Rabies, Lyme Disease, Hanta Virus

and other animal-borne human diseases
in the United States and Canada

*What every Parent, Householder, Camper, Hiker,
Teacher, Wildlife Rehabilitator, Hunter and Fisherman
Needs to Know*

E. Lendell Cockrum, PhD

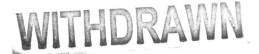

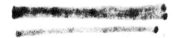

Publishers: Bill Fisher
                     Helen Fisher
                     Howard Fisher

Editor: Bill Fisher

Managing Editor: Sarah Trotta

Book Design: Randy Schultz

Cover Design: Randy Schultz

Published by Fisher Books
4239 W. Ina Road, Suite 101
Tucson, Arizona 85741
(520) 744-6110

Printed in U.S.A.
10 9 8 7 6 5 4 3 2 1

Contents

About the Author

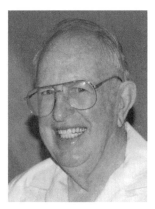

E. Lendell Cockrum, PhD

E. Lendell Cockrum, PhD, has lifelong hands-on experience with mammals and the diseases they carry. His first paper on bats was published in 1939. After returning from the service and coming to Arizona, he was responsible for banding more than 200,000 bats in studies of migrations of the Mexican Free-Tailed Bat. Bats banded in central Arizona were recovered, often just days later, in Mexico as far south as Sinaloa.

A Bachelor of Education graduate from Southern Illinois Normal University, he majored in Zoology with a Botany minor. He obtained his Ph.D. in Zoology from the University of Kansas with an Entomology minor.

His first job out of college was with the U.S. Public Health Service as a Mosquito Control Inspector on a malaria-control project. His active duty in the U.S. Navy included a stint in the Hospital Corps Epidemiology School at the U.S. Naval Hospital in Bethesda, Maryland, and subsequent field experience in Japan. From 1956-1960 he was Consulting Mammalogist with the U. S. Public Health Service, Communicable Disease Center, studying bat rabies.

In 1973-1974 he was a Desert Ecologist Consultant to Massachusetts Institute of Technology in Cambridge, Massachusetts. There he served on a US AID project: Multi-disciplinary development of a framework for evaluating long-term strategies for the development of the Sahel-Sudan Region.

From 1977-1985 he headed the Ecology and Evolutionary Biology Department at the University of Arizona in Tucson. Since 1984 he has been a consulting editor for Encyclopedia Americana. Although he officially retired in 1985, he has continued to write and to be involved in his various interests. Since 1988 he has been a Research Associate for The Museum, Texas Tech University at Lubbock, Texas.

Cockrum's more than 150 publications include 10 books: *Mammals of Kansas, Mammals of Arizona, Mammals of the Southwest, Mammals of the Southwest and Northern New Mexico, Mammals of California and Nevada, Manual of Mammalogy, Biology* (textbook), *Introduction to Mammalogy* (textbook), *Zoology* (textbook), and *Colossal Cave—the Evolution of an Oater*.

Some ABCs of Safety First

*A*lways have some knowledge about the dangers involved in your activities.

*B*e aware of any epidemic (widespread and/or local) animal-borne diseases currently active in the area where you live or where you plan to go hiking, camping or fishing. Remember, a disease may be restricted to a small area or even absent in a given region for months or years and be followed by a serious outbreak.

Where do you find out what animal-borne diseases are active? The local news media (newspapers, television, radio) report many current outbreaks. For additional information, call your local, county, state and provincial health officials, state, provincial and federal game and fish agencies, and park naturalists.

Animal-borne disease epidemics are unusual, but even when there's no outbreak, you should follow normal precautions in dealing with wild animals, whether near your home or during an outdoor activity. If officials are warning about a particular disease, check Table 1 to determine the most common routes of transmission. When you go outdoors, take along any special mosquito, tick or mite repellents needed—as well as any special clothing recommended.

Table 1

Precautions to Avoid Exposure to Animal-Borne Diseases in the United States and Canada

SOURCE OF DISEASE EXPOSURE	DISEASE	SPECIAL PRECAUTIONS
Bite or scratch by infected mammal	Rabies, rabbit fever, tularemia, most others	The most important precaution is to avoid disease-bearing animals and do everything to avoid being scratched or bitten by them. If you are bitten, clean the wound with soap and water; save the mammal for laboratory testing to see what diseases it carries. (Iced or frozen animal material is OK.) Report for medical treatment immediately.
Contact with body fluids of infected mammal (blood, saliva, urine, fecal wastes)	Plague, rabbit fever, rabies, hanta virus, Lyme disease, others	Same as for being bitten or scratched. Not only should you avoid contact with animal fluids (don't skin a dead bobcat with plague for the "rug"), but remember that the ectoparasites (fleas, lice, mites, ticks) are seeking a new warm body.
Bite by infected arthropod		Here are some basic methods of avoiding being bitten and some postexposure suggestions.

Table 1 *continued*

SOURCE OF DISEASE EXPOSURE	DISEASE	SPECIAL PRECAUTIONS
Tick	Lyme disease, Colorado tick fever, Rocky Mountain spotted fever, relapsing fever, ehrlichiosis, babesiosis, tularemia, rabbit fever	Wear clothing that reduces exposure of skin to ticks (pants legs stuffed in socks, long sleeves, etc.). In most areas, druggists can recommend powders or sprays that act as repellents. Your dog is a good collector of ticks. After exposure, examine yourself, children and pets for ticks. Any that have attached should be carefully removed, uncrushed and with mouth parts attached (and not left in your skin!). Accomplish this by grasping the tick (with tweezers) near the mouth parts and pulling upward gently. Insert a needle in your skin, below the tick's mouth parts. Pry out the tick. Disinfect the bite immediately.
Kissing bug	Chagas' disease	In tropics and subtropics, kissing bugs thrive in adobe and thatch buildings as well as in rock walls. In the southwestern United States, they're often found in pack-rat dens in summer cabins. Some humans have extreme allergic reactions to bites, as well as possible exposure to Chagas' disease. Use an insect spray in crevices and other daytime haunts.

Table 1 *continued*

SOURCE OF DISEASE EXPOSURE	DISEASE	SPECIAL PRECAUTIONS
Mosquito	Encephalitis	Use repellents. Ask your druggist about currently available products. In severely infested areas, use mosquito netting over sleeping areas.
Flea	Murine typhus, plague	Fleas from wild animals, dead or alive, often end up on dogs or humans. Various flea powders and sprays are available. Check with your druggist.
Louse	Relapsing fever	Same as for fleas.
Mite (chigger)	Rickettsial pox	Mites are so small that they usually escape notice until they burrow under the skin. They often cling to the tips of grasses and other vegetation, transferring their attention to you as you pass by. The antitick clothing and repellent recommendations are useful. After exposure, washing with soap and water and changing clothes help. Once a mite has burrowed into the skin, treatment to kill the mite is recommended. A paste of baking soda and water or calamine lotion applied to the site may work.

Table 1 *continued*

SOURCE OF DISEASE EXPOSURE	DISEASE	SPECIAL PRECAUTIONS
Contaminated water	Intestinal bacteria, diarrhea, giardiasis, leptospirosis, hanta virus, tularemia, beaver fever, Weil's Syndrome, rabbit fever	Bring your own safe water, or boil or treat unknown water with chemicals. Stagnant water is generally riskier than that in clear flowing streams.
Contaminated food	Intestinal bacteria, diarrhea, hanta virus	Store your food in wild-animal-proof containers.
Contaminated air	Valley fever (coccidiomycosis) and perhaps hanta virus histoplasmosis,	Cleaning rodent nests and wastes from barns and summer cabins helps eliminate the sources of some virus dangers. Fungus spores are often found in dust from soils around rodent dens and barnyards. In rare cases, plague and viral diseases have been contracted by breathing air contaminated by sick or dead animals, especially in confined spaces.

Common sense should guide your actions in dealing with wild mammals and other animals, even when no disease alert has been issued.

Don't attempt to capture that pretty little chipmunk. It's very different from your cuddly pet kitten or puppy. Wild animals are *wild* and they interpret any human approach as dangerous. They react by biting, scratching, and otherwise attacking to protect themselves or attempt to get away.

Watch wild animals—even small ones—from a distance and leave them alone. The seemingly "tame" ones that have learned to take peanuts from your fingers will bite viciously if you try to pick them up. If you hide the peanut in your hand, chipmunks and other rodents have been known to bite in their effort to reach the food.

Every wild mammal has a normal pattern of behavior. If you see one acting in an unusual way (a bat lying on the ground, a chipmunk that permits you to pick it up, and so on), it is probably sick. While it may be affected by a condition that can't be transmitted to humans, you won't be able to determine this.

Don't take chances. If for some reason it's necessary for you to handle a sick or dead animal, use precautions to ensure that body fluids of the sick animal don't contaminate you or your clothing. The only reason you could have for handling an animal in the wild is if it has bitten or otherwise touched someone and you need to have it tested to see if it carries any disease.

Finally, remember that almost all the diseases described in this book (especially those of rodents and rabbits) infect humans by accident, not because of the animal's behavior. Most such accidental infections result when humans invade the normal habitat of the wild animal and encounter its parasites and diseases. Less commonly, wild animals (especially rats and mice) invade homes, barns, or neighborhoods. Thus, each of these diseases could, theoretically, be contracted by a human being who has never left his or her 20th-floor Main Street apartment in Downtown, U.S.A. or Canada. After all, animals don't recognize that we consider our buildings to be ours, not theirs. It's always the responsibility of the human being to exercise precaution against animal-borne diseases.

Diseases Associated with Bats, Rodents and Rabbits

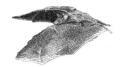

Every few weeks, it seems the news media report another case (or series of cases) of people contracting a disease associated with bats, rodents, or rabbits. In the past few years, Lyme disease and hanta virus have been much publicized. An apparent recent increase in the number of children exposed to bats resulted in several warnings to schools and teachers from public health and wildlife management officials about the dangers of bat rabies. Of special concern are children in the lower grades who are noted for picking up strange animals for "Show and Tell."

For most of us, both the disease and the animal involved are mysteries.

In late 1996, an Associated Press report appeared under the title: "Australia Names Bats Hosts of Deadly Virus." Apparently another bat-borne virus affecting horses and humans has been added to the growing list of animal-borne human diseases. This one is caused by *Morbillivirus,* a relative of the viruses causing human measles, dog distemper and cattle plague. To date, it is known to have caused death in several horses and in two horse trainers. Death resulted from rapid, massive degeneration of lung tissues—somewhat reminiscent of the effects of the hanta virus carried by rodents.

The means of transmission of this new disease has not been determined. Is the virus airborne? Could humans and horses be acquiring it by direct contact with bats, through saliva, or via contaminated food or water? The question is complicated by the fact that the bat host is one of the flying foxes that feeds only on fruits and blossoms, and thus has little direct contact with horses or humans.

The mysterious *Ebola* virus of tropical Africa is another disease that continues to receive publicity in the United States. Neither the reservoir (the host animal on which the virus makes its home) nor the means of transmission of this deadly virus has yet been identified. So far, extensive testing of rodents has failed to prove anything. One report suggests that bats may be the reservoir but no proof yet exists.

This book has been assembled for those interested in animal-borne diseases that can affect humans in the United States and Canada. It contains information useful to the concerned lay reader as well as to health professionals and animal-control technicians.

It's written to help avid hunters, fishermen, campers, hikers, and others who enjoy the outdoors pursue their activities more safely. It also contains information helpful to homeowners who are concerned about exposure to rodents, bats or rabbits in their residences or outlying property. In addition, parents and pet owners may find this an informative, reassuring guide.

This book is a primer. As such, like all ABC books, it presents a simple overview of the subject. For further information, you may wish to examine some of the sources listed in the reference section. For accurate information on treating animal-borne illnesses, consult your medical doctor. For more advice about controlling animals, contact a professional such as a pest-control service, agricultural extension agent, or state or federal fish and wildlife service personnel.

～

Human diseases are generally divided into a number of types, based primarily on cause (for example, infectious diseases, nutritional diseases, circulatory diseases, mental diseases and others). Infectious diseases are those caused by contact with various organisms. Human infectious diseases are usually subdivided into infectious diseases (those caused by viruses, rickettsias, bacteria or fungi) and parasitic diseases (those caused by protozoans or helminths—intestinal worms).

Here we're concerned with the infectious diseases that people and domesticated animals can acquire from bats, rodents, and rabbits. When the causative organism of a disease is normally found in the bat, rodent, or rabbit, the animal is termed a *reservoir*. The infectious organism doesn't always cause the host animal to become ill but can make other animals and people sick.

The disease-causing organisms reach humans in various ways, differing from disease to disease. You can pick up an animal-borne disease by consuming food and water contaminated with the organism. Other organisms, especially viruses and spores of fungi, may be airborne, infecting humans who inhale them. Still others can't infect humans until they enter the bloodstream. Open sores and wounds, bites and scratches on a person's skin can all serve as infection routes.

Being bitten by a tick, mite or insect (flea, louse, mosquito, kissing bug) that has been feeding on an infected animal can also transmit the infection to you. Such transmitters are known as *vectors*.

Diagram 1 summarizes some of the primary ways in which animal-borne diseases reach humans.

Diagram 1. Possible routes of diseases from bats, rodents, or rabbits to humans.

Saliva	▶ ——————— **CONTACT** ——————— ▶	Human
Breath	▶ ——————— **AIR** ——————— ▶	

	▶ ————— **BITE** ————— ▶	
	ARTHROPOD VECTORS	
	▶ ——— Tick ——— ▶	
Rat	▶ ——— Kissing Bug ——— ▶	Human
	▶ ——— Mosquito ——— ▶	
	▶ ——— Flea ——— ▶	
	▶ ——— Louse ——— ▶	
	▶ ——— Mite (chigger) ——— ▶	

Urine	▶ ——— House Fly ——— ▶	Human
and	**CONTAMINATION**	Food and
Droppings	▶ ——————————— ▶	Water

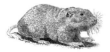 Some disease-causing organisms can be transmitted by more than one route. For example, if you handle a sick or dead diseased animal you can be infected through a scratch in your skin. You can also be infected through the bite of a live animal or of some vector carrying the organism. Some viruses can be spread by contact, by breathing or by eating or drinking contaminated food or water. Dirty hands can contaminate food or water as well as directly infect the human.

Given all the ways people can acquire animal-borne diseases, you may wonder why more people aren't infected much more often. In fact, despite the publicity some outbreaks receive, human contraction of such diseases is still pretty uncommon.

Several interacting factors make this true. First, healthy humans (and healthy animals) can usually overcome a very light "infection." In fact, the vaccines used for human protection against some diseases (e.g., polio, Rocky Mountain spotted fever) are made from live or dead disease organisms.

Another factor that protects us from animal-borne diseases is that not all organisms of a given kind are equally virulent. Infections from some populations of disease-causing organisms (those occupying a particular area) may be very minor, while others of the same species may cause extreme sickness and even death. Just what causes this variation is not fully understood. Part of the answer depends on how many of the infective organisms are involved.

The resistance of the infected person is another variable. A strong, healthy person can often recover more quickly than someone whose physical condition is already weakened by such conditions as stress, starvation, injury or the effects of another disease. That's why you often hear that infectious diseases are particularly dangerous to the elderly, young children or those in poor health.

Still another protective factor is that, at most times, infected bats, rodents or rabbits are extremely rare. In fact, a recent newspaper account reported that in the attempt to isolate

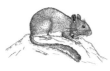 the *Hanta virus,* a total of 19,000 sample animals had been studied before the virus was located.

But exposure does occur, and some people are infected by animal-borne diseases. Some of these diseases can make you quite sick or even be fatal, so it isn't wise to count on natural protections alone. Common sense is your best ally against infection. Obviously, you shouldn't go around deliberately exposing yourself to infections of any sort! Any time you see a wild animal under abnormal conditions, assume that it's probably sick. Wild animals in their own habitats should be left alone.

That "cute little chipmunk" that young Johnny was able to catch while on the class picnic was probably sick. Whether it suffered from some disease that could be transmitted to Johnny isn't clear from looking at the animal, but why take a chance? If the chipmunk was healthy enough to bite Johnny in its attempt to escape his clutches, you'll face another dilemma. If the chipmunk has escaped, it can't be tested for diseases. Most likely Johnny's doctor will advise that he have rabies shots just to be on the safe side. Even though rabies in rodents is extremely rare, no one wants to take even a remote chance that this chipmunk was the exception.

Even dead animals can be dangerous to humans. A few years ago, a college student—a newcomer to the Southwest—found a bobcat that had been run over on a highway just outside of town. "Aha!," he thought, "a bobcat rug for my dormitory room!" Not knowing the bobcat was infected with the plague, the student began skinning the animal. When he became ill, he was fortunate enough to be treated by doctors who were aware of the presence of plague in the region. He had only a mild case.

What if the student had been a visitor from a large eastern city? What if, upon returning home a week or so later, he became ill? Would the doctor have quickly thought of plague? Or would the doctor have been baffled as to the cause of the illness?

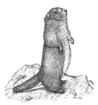 The basic advice of this book is: *Avoid touching any sick or dead animal without taking proper precautions. And never let a child be unnecessarily exposed to sick or dead wild animals.*

The early symptoms of many animal-borne infections are similar. They usually include flulike features: The onset is often sudden, with chills and fevers (usually over 100.5F, 38C), aches and pains (in the head, muscles, or joints) and often fatigue and weakness. All these discomforts result from the body's reaction to the rapidly increasing population of the invading organism (whether a virus, rickettsia, bacterium or protozoan). These organisms secrete poisons and alert the human's immune system to fight them. Those poisons, and the products released by the dead organisms killed by the body's defense system, make you sick.

This book can help you identify disease-carrying animals and understand how they can lead to infectious human illnesses. It also contains advice on what to do if you are exposed to an animal-borne disease.

The material is presented in three sections.

First is a brief overview of the more common bat-, rodent- and rabbit-borne diseases that occur in the United States and Canada. Some of these diseases also occur in other parts of the world. And other countries have animal-borne diseases that, luckily, haven't yet made their way to this region. For example, the United States and Canada haven't been affected by scrub typhus (tsutsugamushi fever), which is caused by a species of Rickettsia and transmitted by chiggers, and has infected humans in Asia.

The second section of this book introduces the ecology and biology of the various bats, rodents, and rabbits of the world. These pages introduce the reader to the habitats, distribution, diet, activities and adaptations of these mammals.

The third section contains brief descriptions, distribution maps, drawings and photographs of the major types of bats, rodents and rabbits of the United States and Canada that have been involved in cases of animal-borne diseases of humans. The animal descriptions, and accompanying maps and illustrations, provide ways to identify the "guilty critters."

The book ends with a short list of references that are available in larger public libraries.

Most Common Diseases

*M*ost of the publicized animal-borne diseases derive primarily from three groups of mammals: bats, rodents and rabbits. Public health agencies have focused on these diseases and attempted to eradicate them.

However, as you read about these diseases it's important to remember that many human infectious and parasitic diseases don't involve bats, rodents or rabbits as reservoirs or intermediate hosts. Several are transmitted from one human to another, often without even an arthropod vector. Arthropods are insects and other simple animals with jointed bodies and limbs, such as the mosquito, fly and chigger. Most, but not all, are insects.

Also keep in mind that animals besides bats, rodents, and rabbits can be disease reservoirs. Diseases in which animals serve as reservoirs are termed *zoonoses* (singular, zoonosis). Those that are present at all times in a small number of animals are termed *enzootic* (endemic) diseases; those that affect a large number of animals in a given region, all within a short time, are termed *epizootic* (epidemic) diseases.

In addition, bats, rodents and rabbits are subject to various infections that aren't transmitted to humans. Thus, a sick animal doesn't necessarily present a threat to humans.

The diseases explored in this book are the major zoonoses found in the United States in which bats, rodents or rabbits are primary or partial reservoirs. Most human cases result when a causative organism is transmitted from an animal to a human via a vector. A few of these diseases, such as the plague, can also be transmitted by various means from one human directly to another.

Obviously, one certain way for humans to escape these diseases is to avoid infection. However, by accident, necessity or desire, we may come into contact with bats, rodents or rabbits, their contaminated areas or their potential vectors, such as ticks and fleas. And we may be exposed to the diseases they carry. Because these diseases are transmitted by microorganisms sometimes not visible even with a microscope, it's impossible to know when you're near them. It's also very difficult to see insect vectors and animal habitats before you're in contact with them. Therefore, general precautions to protect yourself, your children and pets are essential.

In the past, heroic efforts have been made to exterminate all of the reservoir mammals in an area as a means of eliminating disease reservoirs. Such plague reservoirs as Old World rats (Norway and black), house mice, prairie dogs and ground squirrels have all been targets of these programs. Usually these efforts have resulted in a temporary, local reduction in populations at best. These mammals have a way of coming back.

Health officials have also attacked arthropod vectors. One approach involves controlling mosquitoes and spraying insecticides into rodent burrows to kill ticks and fleas. These programs have been locally successful for short times. Most such programs are not only of limited effectiveness but are extremely expensive. Thus, they're usually attempted only during epidemics.

These control measures bring dangers of their own. Not only do disease organisms generally resist them, but humans and domestic animals can be harmed by the chemicals used in the control attempt.

Although we don't yet have a safe, effective way to eliminate animal-borne human diseases, there are steps you can take to reduce the danger of infection. Just as driving a safer car, maintaining a reasonable speed and wearing a seat belt help you reduce your chance of being killed in an automobile accident, you can reduce your risk of infection from animal-borne diseases, even when you're in an area where these diseases are known to exist. As Table 1 shows, you can avoid vectors by using insect repellents and wearing protective clothing. Taking care about personal cleanliness and being sure you consume only clean food and water are other helpful precautions.

Knowing what animals you've been exposed to can also be important. As you'll read, many of these diseases are serious, sometimes even fatal, so recognizing the animals that you've been in contact with can help doctors begin the correct treatment right away, perhaps even saving a life. In some cases you can bring the infective animal to the doctor with you to be tested for exactly what diseases it carries.

What diseases do you need to protect yourself from? This chapter groups them by causative organisms: viruses, rickettsias, bacteria, protozoa and fungi.

Table 2

Infectious Diseases (Caused by Viruses, Rickettsia, Bacteria, Fungi) and Parasitic Diseases (Caused by Protozoans)

DISEASE	CAUSATIVE ORGANISM	MAJOR RESERVOIR	TRANSMISSION
Colorado Tick Fever	Arbovirus	Ground Squirrel	Ticks
Encephalitis	Arbovirus	Rodents	Mosquitoes
Hanta Virus Pulmonary Syndrome	Hanta virus	Deer Mouse	and perhaps Air Contact
Dengue	Virus	Rodents and Birds	Mosquitoes
Rabies	Rhabdovirus	Rodents (Minor)	Bites
Rickettsial Pox	Rickettsia	House Mouse & Old World Rats	Mite
Murine Typhus	Rickettsia	Rodents	Fleas
Rocky Mountain Spotted Fever	Rickettsia	Rodents	Ticks
Ehrlichiosis	Rickettsia	?	Ticks
Intestinal Bacteria	Bacterium	Rodents (Minor)	Contamination
Leptospirosis	Bacterium	Rodents (plus other mammals)	Animal urine
Lyme Disease	Bacterium	Rodents (plus other mammals)	Ticks
Plague	Bacterium	Rodents	Fleas
Relapsing Fever	Bacterium	Rodents	Ticks, Lice
Tularemia	Bacterium	Rodents (plus other mammals)	Deer Fly Contact
Babesiosis	Protozoan	Rodents	Ticks
Chagas' Disease	Protozoan	Rodents	Kissing Bug
Giardiasis	Protozoan	Beaver	Water
Coccidiomycosis (Valley Fever)	Fungus	Rodent Burrows	Air
Histoplasmosis	Fungus	Soil, Caves	Air

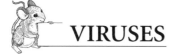 # VIRUSES

Viruses are extremely tiny organisms that are smaller than bacteria. Most aren't visible with most microscopes. They reproduce only in the cell of some plant or animal, a process that causes a disease. Viruses can transmit diseases to humans in a number of ways: A person can breathe in some viruses; others get into the bloodstream through the bite of a reservoir animal or vector. In some cases, just touching an infected wild animal or pet may allow the virus to get in through body openings. Contact with a carrier animal's saliva or other fluids can also transmit viruses in those fluids.

Because virus infections cannot be successfully controlled by antibiotics or other available medicines, the usual treatment is *symptomatic*—treating the symptoms. This may involve reducing the patient's activities (bed rest or even hospital care), controlling the fever (medication and even cold-water or alcohol washes, increasing fluid intake (in severe cases, the use of intravenously administered fluids) and control of pain and/or coughing (medication).

Five of the most common virus-caused human/animal diseases in the United States are: hanta virus pulmonary syndrome, Colorado tick fever, encephalitis (five varieties), dengue and rabies.

Hanta Virus Pulmonary Syndrome (HPS)

For years, the term "ARDS" (adult respiratory distress syndrome) has been used to describe a form of severe breathing difficulty that leads to serious illness and death in human beings. The causes of this syndrome have been unclear, and most medical experts think there are many causes of ARDS. Generally, ARDS deaths are attributed to unknown causes that resulted in extreme respiratory distress.

Since May 1993, some ARDS cases have been recognized as being caused by a *Hanta virus,* a virus in the family Bunyaviridae. This form of ARDS has been given several names: "hanta virus"—from the causative organism, "Four Corners disease"—from the geographic area in the Southwest where it was first diagnosed, and "hanta virus pulmonary syndrome"—from the symptoms in humans affecting their lungs, and even "mystery disease."

By February 1994, at least 52 cases (31 of them fatal) had been reported of a previously unknown hanta virus that affected the lungs. These cases occurred in 13 states west of the Mississippi River (mostly in the Southwest), plus one case in Florida and one in Rhode Island. Because it has been recorded in North Dakota, probably some of the ARDS (Adult Respiratory Distress Syndrome) cases in the Canadian Prairie Provinces were actually hanta virus. The hanta virus pulmonary syndrome virus has also been called the "Muerto Canyon virus," from Canyon del Muerto (Canyon of Death) on the Apache Indian Reservation in northeastern Arizona, a site near the point of origin of the first diagnosed case in 1993. In hindsight, it appears that an August 1991 case in North Dakota was actually the first certain case of the "new" hanta virus. Not only were the symptoms similar, but some tissue samples of the victims appear to test positive for this virus.

Other types of hanta virus infections, associated with kidney malfunctions rather than respiratory problems, had been identified earlier, almost all in the eastern hemisphere, mainly Europe and Asia. Four different types had been identified: Hantaan, Seoul, Puumala, and Prospect Hill. All involve rodents as reservoirs. The names are drawn from the geographic areas where the virus was first identified: Hantaan River, China; Seoul, Korea; Puumala, Sweden; and Prospect Hill, Pennsylvania. The latter variety was isolated from rodents in the mid-1980s but isn't known to cause a disease in humans.

In response to the outbreak of the lung-affecting hanta virus cases in the summer and fall of 1993, the U.S. Public Health Service's Centers for Disease Control and Prevention (CDC) undertook a major effort to learn how to control the disease. Some state health departments were also involved.

Their studies found that incubation time—the period between exposure to the virus and detectable disease symptoms—ranges from one to five weeks. Early symptoms of this form of ARDS are flulike, including a cough, fever (over 100F, 37.8C), aches, and pains. Some surviving patients report that the onset was mild. One reported first feeling "feverish, nauseated, and sleepy."

One man had a slight cough and an upset stomach for some days before he developed chills and fever reaching 103F (39.5C). Treatment with antibiotics for one week was useless. During this time he developed unusual behavior; he didn't know where he was or whether it was day or night. He was hospitalized with fluid filling the lungs and very low blood pressure. Eventually he improved.

By contrast, several of those who died from hanta virus pulmonary syndrome appear to have had a rapid onset, with only a few hours between first symptoms and death.

To date, the scientists studying this new disease have found most cases to be associated with the deer mouse, *Peromyscus maniculatus*. But laboratory tests show that the closely related *Peromyscus boylii* (brush mouse) and *Peromyscus truei* (piñon mice), as well as chipmunks, wood rats and house mice, are carriers of the disease. Further studies will probably enlarge the list to include most native rats and mice as well as most members of the squirrel family.

Of the deer mice, *Peromyscus maniculatus* is the kind most apt to enter human buildings, such as houses and barns. These mice are widespread in rural areas but rare in urban areas. Because it is found in such a wide range, this species has been pinpointed as the major potential danger to humans. However, people in any out-of-doors situation may contact this or other species of rodents and, perhaps, be exposed to the hanta virus.

Recent attention to this relatively new animal-borne disease has revealed some helpful information. But a number of questions remain to be answered, including:

1. Is the virus a newcomer to North America, or has it been around for a long time?
   Doctors recognize that there are multiple causes for ARDS. Many people die of unexplained pulmonary syndromes every year. Probably some of these cases were actually the result of hanta virus.

2. Is it possible that the disease is endemic to the New World (the western hemisphere, mainly North and South America) but is only now being recognized?

According to newspaper reports, some nonbiologists contend that the disease was introduced into the United States in World War II as a result of undocumented biological warfare. Still others claim the virus is an "escapee" from some later governmental experiment in biological warfare. Neither of these "theories" appears logical or probable.

3. Is the current "outbreak" the result of a harmless type of the virus being made dangerous by mutation? Or could it be caused by an increase in rodent populations resulting from heavy rains?

4. Is the deer mouse the only reservoir?

Recent tests indicate that at least three species of Peromyscus, some ground squirrels, a wood rat and a chipmunk are possible reservoirs. Are other species of rodents also reservoirs?

5. Is the disease likely to become an urban as well as a rural problem?

A recent report of a positive test on a house mouse suggests that certain rats and mice (house mice, black rats and Norway rats) may serve as reservoirs. These rodents are more common in cities than the type known to carry the virus.

6. Do mild, undiagnosed cases occur?

7. How does the virus affect the rodent that transmits it?

Some studies indicate that carrier rodents appear to be well and to have a normal life span. They may have developed antibodies to resist the disease. Transmission of the hanta virus pulmonary syndrome virus to other rodents (and to humans) appears to be through contact with rodent urine, saliva and fecal material.

8. How long is the Hanta virus infectious after it is outside the body of the rodent?

One investigator stated: "When the virus is exposed to sunlight, it dies within a few minutes." However, rodent-contaminated debris is often suspected as the source of human infections, indicating that the virus may live—and be dangerous to people much longer than was believed.

Colorado Tick Fever (CTF)

This disease is known to be caused when a human is infected by the *Coltivirus,* which is one of a group of viruses called an "arbovirus" (an arthropod-borne virus). Colorado tick fever is transmitted by ticks, an arthropod of the genus *Dermacentor,* from a reservoir rodent to a human. The tick bites the rodent, acquiring the virus in its saliva, then bites the person, transmitting the virus into the bloodstream.

Both Colorado tick fever and Rocky Mountain spotted fever were first recognized in 1859. Both were formerly called *mountain fever* and weren't recognized as separate diseases until the late 1800s. (As you'll see in a later section, Rocky Mountain spotted fever is caused by a rickettsia organism, not a virus.)

Most cases of Colorado tick fever are found in the mountains of the western United States and Canada. Some 200 to 300 cases are reported each year, but some experts think that most cases are unreported. Most infections are contracted between late May and early July.

Incubation in humans is usually four to six days following a tick bite. Symptoms include chills and fever (to 104F, 40C), severe headache, sensitivity to bright lights, aches and pains in muscles and joints (especially in the lower back) and often, nausea and loss of appetite. After about six days the symptoms clear up, only to reappear one or sometimes two times at intervals of two or three days. Untreated, recovery is usually rapid. However, severe complications do sometimes occur.

Ground squirrels appear to be the major reservoir for the Colorado tick fever virus, but the organism has also been found in rabbits, marmots, voles and porcupines.

Encephalitis

Encephalitis is an inflammation of the brain, in humans and in other animals, that can be caused by several different factors. One of the most frequent forms is brain inflammations caused by any of several togaviruses.

These arboviruses are usually transmitted by mosquitoes, but some are known to be transmitted by ticks. They occur in many parts of the world, including Australia, Africa, Asia,

Europe, South America and North America. The natural reservoir is generally one or more kinds of birds, but several mammals, including rabbits and rodents, have been found infected.

In humans, some varieties of viral encephalitis cause only mild symptoms and soon clear up, even without treatment. Other cases are severe, even fatal, in their effects. Incubation is usually four to six days following the bite of an infected mosquito. Early symptoms include headaches, fever (to 104F, 40C), and pain and weakness in the muscles. After about two days, the symptoms usually clear up, only to sometimes reappear once or twice at intervals of two or three days.

In the this area, six different types of encephalitis, caused by related viruses, are recognized. Outbreaks among domestic animals and humans occur mainly in the spring and summer, often following rainy seasons when mosquito populations are high. Sometimes horses and mules are given vaccinations against one or more of the varieties.

Eastern equine encephalitis (EEE) is most common in horses and mules in the eastern United States and Canada. In addition to birds, cottontails and rodents have been implicated as reservoirs. This is often a fatal disease in humans.

Venezuelan equine encephalitis (VEE) is more common in Central and South America but outbreaks have occurred in the southeastern United States from Florida to Texas. It was first recognized in 1935 from cases in Venezuela. Again, birds are the main reservoir, but cottontails and rodents are also involved. It is generally a mild disease in people.

Western equine encephalitis (WEE) occurs mainly west of the Mississippi River. It, too, is usually mild in humans.

California encephalitis (CE) has been isolated from tree squirrels and ground squirrels as well as opossums. It occurs occasionally in humans.

La Crosse encephalitis (LCE) first recognized in La Crosse, Wisconsin, is similar to California Encephalitis. It is transmitted from the rodent reservoit to humans by the kind of mosquito that develops in water in holes in trees and other small amounts of water such as in tin cans and old tires. More than 2000 cases were reported between 1964 (when first recognized) and 1997. Some cases in children have resulted in permanent brain damage.

St. Louis encephalitis (SLE) is similar to western equine encephalitis. It was first observed in 1932 among human patients in St. Louis, Missouri.

Causative viruses of encephalitis have been isolated from cottontail rabbits, ground squirrels, chipmunks, tree squirrels, cotton rats and kangaroo rats.

Dengue (Breakbone Fever)

Dengue is a viral disease typically found in tropical and subtropical regions, especially Southeast Asia, Japan, Australia, Central and South America, and various Caribbean islands. Dengue (pronounced DEN-gie) is transmitted by *Aedes egypti* mosquitoes, a species that occurs in many of the tropical and subtropical parts of the world.

Two to four days after having been infected, human victims suffer from a sudden fever and severe headaches, followed a few days later by sore eyes, sore throat and a reddish rash. This is often followed by severe pains in the muscles, back and joints, thus the name, *breakbone fever.* The fever usually drops after about a week.

This discomfort is followed by a recovery period of about two weeks, characterized by loss of appetite and general malaise (just not feeling good). Treatment for dengue consists of bed rest, fluids and painkillers, usually aspirin.

Scattered cases have been diagnosed in the United States and Canada, including a man in New England who became ill after his return from a trip to the Caribbean. About 50 cases occurred in U.S. troops after a tour of duty in Haiti. A minor outbreak took place in south Texas in 1995, across the border from a major outbreak in Tamaulipas, Mexico. Of the 29 cases diagnosed in Texas, 14 of the people had recently visited Mexico.

Because *Aedes egypti* mosquitoes are found in the southern parts of the United States, it's possible that the disease is being introduced into native birds and rodents from Americans returning home from an infected area. In these areas, the mosquitoes are usually inactive during the winter months, restricting the possibility of epidemics. Outbreaks occur only in the warmer summer months.

Rabies

Rabies is perhaps the best-known animal-borne disease, and one that adults and children have learned to fear. Untreated, it's fatal to humans, dogs and cats, as well as other animals. Who can forget the movie "Old Yeller" or many popular stories of beloved animals and children suffering and dying from rabies?

It's caused by a *Rhabdovirus,* a type of virus named for its rodlike shape. Scientists are just beginning to identify various viruses within this species that transmit different forms of rabies. Apparently any mammal can be infected. Cows, horses, sheep, goats, rabbits and rodents are all known to be susceptible. However, dogs, cats, wild carnivores (especially skunks, coyotes, foxes and raccoons), and bats make up the major reservoir. Some medical technicians list rodents, rabbits, and other "nonbiting" animals such as deer and livestock, as "dead-end hosts," meaning they can contract the virus but they don't generally transmit it because they don't bite other animals. One assumes humans would also be classified as "dead-end hosts!"

Kangaroo rats, cotton rats, flying squirrels, voles and other rodents have been proven to be highly or extremely susceptible to lethal rabies infections. Several rabid groundhogs (also called *marmots* or *woodchucks*) are detected each year. All can transmit the virus to humans.

Rabies is usually transmitted to a person or another animal by the bite of an infected animal, with the saliva containing the virus. However, a number of rabies deaths have been reported in which no animal bite was recorded. Such "cryptic rabies" cases are usually assumed to be the result of contaminated saliva or other body fluids of the infected animal having entered the person's body by way of a scratch in the skin or even through moist tissues such as the lip or eye.

Once in the host, the rhabdovirus makes it way to a nerve, then travels along nerves to the brain where it multiplies and leads to full-blown disease. Cases that aren't treated before the virus enters the nervous system are usually fatal. If given shortly after exposure, a series of immunization shots is generally effective in preventing the disease.

Unfortunately, none of the current treatments can arrest or eliminate rabies that has a "proper" incubation period and has begun to multiply. The length of this period varies greatly. Laboratory experiments with various animals reveal that it may vary from a few days to months—even a year or more.

Early symptoms are much like those of other infections—fever, a general sick feeling, head and muscle aches, depression and swelling of the lymph nodes. Once the virus enters the nervous system, symptoms may include confusion, irrational behavior and muscle spasms—especially in those muscles that control breathing and swallowing. Even the sight of water may cause increased spasms. Death usually occurs 3 to 6 days after severe symptoms develop.

Thus, people who have been exposed to rabies (as determined by a laboratory test on the sick animal), or bitten by an escaped animal whose status is unknown, are given the series of rabies treatment shots almost as soon as they make their way from the waiting room into the doctor's office.

The good news about rabies is that effective vaccinations are available, both for humans and pets. Antirabies vaccinations for dogs are now essentially as routine as buying the dog's food, and are required by law in most states. However, pet cats that go outdoors are just as likely to contact a wild, rabid animal or pet as are dogs. So far, most cat owners don't have their cats vaccinated.

Just how many cases of rabies in animals occur each year is not known. The CDC compiles reports from state health laboratories each year. Diagrams 2-4 summarize some of the data concerning the variations of the prevalence of rabies in animals in the United States during three of the last 40 years. Rabies has been isolated from bats taken in central Ontario and western Quebec.

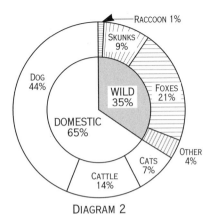

DIAGRAM 2

Type of mammal involved in positive tests for rabies
reported to the United States Public Health Service in 1955
(modified from Brass 1994). Total, 5,450 tested.

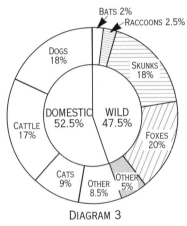

DIAGRAM 3

Type of mammal involved in positive tests
for rabies reported to the United States
Public Health Service in 1960 (modified
from Brass 1954). Total, 3,900 tested.

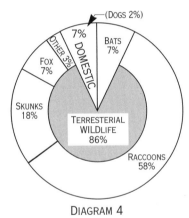

DIAGRAM 4

Type of mammal involved in positive tests
for rabies reported to the United States
Public Health Service in 1994 (modified from
Krebs *et al* 1995). Total, 6,947 tested.

Note that in 1955 the most commonly reported cases were in
domestic mammals, especially dogs. In fact, 47 percent of the
5,700 reported cases occurred in dogs. By 1960, dogs made up
only 18 percent of the 3,900 reported cases. In 1994, less than 2
percent of the positive tests were in dogs.

The difference? In the late 1950s, a successful antirabies vaccine was developed and became a standard requirement for dogs. Over the years, stricter monitoring has made rabies vaccinations for dogs commonplace.

Between 1992 and 1994, a significant outbreak occurred in wild mammals, especially in raccoons (Diagram 3). Many more tests were performed on animals (8,147 in contrast to the 3,900 in 1960). Whether there was a significant increase in the number of humans bitten by rabid animals is unclear. Certainly much of the increase in animal cases was the result of better monitoring by federal and state health laboratories and wildlife managers.

Table 3 summarizes human rabies cases in part of this same period. Note that in the 10-year period of 1950-1959, a total of 113 human deaths resulted from rabies—an average of 11.3 deaths each year. Actually, most of these were in the first five years of this period. The most common probable transmitter was a dog.

Table 3

Cases of Rabies in Humans in the United States, 1950-1989 (Modified from Brass, 1994)

		SOURCE			
Years	Total	domestic	unknown	wild	laboratory
1950-59 (10 years)	113	71	26	14	2
1960-1989 (30 years)	51	23*	12	13	2

Note: The source of the infection is indicated as domestic animal (mainly dogs), unknown, wild mammal, or accidents in laboratories working with live rabies viruses. The * indicates that 14 of the original infections resulted from bites received outside of the United States (see text).

In contrast, after the successful dog antirabies vaccine was developed and usage enforced (mainly by dog-licensing laws), the next 30 years (1960-1989) saw the total human rabies deaths drop to 51—an average of 1.7 each year. In 23 cases, dogs were involved. However, 14 of the 23 actually resulted from dog bites received somewhere outside the United States (Haiti, Mexico, Southeast Asia), with rabies developing when the victim returned to the States.

Even though the number of human deaths from rabies per year is insignificant, the high mortality rate among those who have been infected is certainly cause for alarm. People who are routinely exposed to unvaccinated animals (for example, animal caretakers, rehabilitators, wildlife technicians, animal exterminators) should consult their medical doctors and ask about taking pre-exposure immunization shots.

Rabies is sometimes called *hydrophobia*—fear of water— because victims in terminal stages refuse to drink liquids and react violently in attempts to give them fluids orally. Rabies has been recognized as a disease caused by some transmittable organism since the classical experiments of French chemist Louis Pasteur in the mid-nineteenth century. Pasteur is best known for his pioneering work that resulted in the "pasteurization" process, which is now routine in the processing of milk and various other foods. He also developed the Pasteur treatment for rabies, which was standard for humans exposed to the disease until just a few years ago. Since about 1955, less painful treatments have been available.

While many mammals have been implicated in transmitting rabies, the role of vampire bats in spreading the disease to livestock, wild animals and unprotected humans in the tropics of the New World has also long been recognized. In spite of various efforts to control vampire-bat populations, their presence continues to be a public-health concern as well as a major deterrent to profitable livestock industries in several tropical New World regions.

As early as 1954, it became known that insectivorous bats (those that eat insects) were also reservoirs and transmitters of rabies in the United States and Canada. Recent studies, using new biochemical techniques, reveal that an as-yet-undetermined number of varieties of rabies viruses are present in nature. Thus, a rabies virus isolated from a victim (human or other mammal) can be identified as primarily associated with a given group of mammals.

In this area two major types appear to exist. One persists year after year as a reservoir in wild terrestrial mammals (especially raccoons, skunks, and coyotes). The second is a reservoir in insectivorous bats. Each group has unique minor varieties, thus enabling investigators to determine which kind (or kinds) of wild mammal is the primary source of a particular case.

Many of these findings, especially those about bat rabies in general, are discussed in only a few recent general references. Warrell (1995) presents a brief overview of much of the literature of the past decade. Brass (1994) gives an exhaustive summary.

The early reports are still unclear but it appears that, so far, three minor varieties of the bat rabies virus occur in the United States and Canada: (a) silver-haired bat type; (b) *Myotis* type; and (c) Mexican free-tailed (or guano) bat type. These viruses are named for the type of bat in which they were first isolated. Especially during outbreaks in nature, the viruses "spill over" into other species. For example, the silver-haired bat variety may well be found in some other bat species and in terrestrial wildlife and domestic animals.

Some human deaths have been labeled "cryptic bat rabies" when the victim had no known exposure to bats. In these cases, biochemical evidence clearly indicated that one of the identified bat rabies viruses was involved. Some victims, such as young children or those with poor memory, may have actually been exposed to a bat but were unable to recall the event. Others were probably infected through an encounter with an unvaccinated cat or other domestic animal that had been in contact with a rabid bat. Later the cat, in its normal behavior (licking or play-biting of the human), may well have transmitted the virus, which still carried its biochemical label as bat rabies.

During the past 40 years, every species of bats in the United States and Canada has tested positive for rabies at one time or another. As publicity campaigns have increased public awareness of bat rabies, more and more bats are submitted to state and regional health laboratories for testing.

Most bats submitted for examination were found in some atypical situation—on the ground, in a house, cornered by a cat. That fact leads one to suspect that many may have been sick.

However, others have been caught by humans and brought to labs during periods of migration. Certain bat species make annual migrations from winter to summer habitats. The silver-haired bat, like many humans, normally migrates to Canada for the summer and to the southern United States for the winter. While on these treks, they are often in unfamiliar territory and hang up for the day in a place exposed to human (or pet) observation. During these periods the number of bats submitted for examination increases sharply.

As shown in diagrams 2-4, the total number of positive rabies examinations in bats is low. The numbers submitted for examination are much larger. For example, in New York state, between 1988 and 1992, 6,810 bats were examined, only 4.6 percent of which were positive for rabies (Childs et al., 1994). In Illinois, in a 22-year period (1965-1986), 4,272 bats were examined, of which 6 percent tested positive (Burnett, 1989). Tests of bats taken at random from populations of normal, healthy bats have produced even lower percentages of infected animals.

Some reports and medical advisories have linked cryptic bat rabies to a series of experiments performed in the early 1960s in which bat rabies was transmitted through the air to captive carnivores. In the experiments, carried out in a large cave in Texas, foxes, coyotes and other carnivores were kept in bat-proof cages for up to 30 days. Directly above them was part of a maternity colony of Brazilian free-tailed bats (the same as Mexican free-tailed or guano bats) estimated to contains as many as 20-million females and their young. The experimenters described the place as an "extremely oppressive cave room atmosphere, which was hot, humid and heavily charged with ammonia."

The carnivores were kept in cages that permitted no contact with bats or arthropods. They breathed in hot air, humid from urinary and fecal wastes. Even with no direct contact, some of these animals developed rabies after an incubation period (measured from first day of exposure in the cave) of 28 to 109 days.

Based on these experiments, a news release from the Communicable Diseases Center in Atlanta, Georgia, was published in Time magazine of September 29, 1961. The report, entitled "Beware of Bats" concluded: "Even the noxious air of a bat cave seems to transmit the disease." Shortly thereafter, the CDC issued warnings to State and County Public Health officials that bat rabies had increased greatly since it was first recognized in the 1950s. They warned that humans, even in open air over which a single bat has flown, had been exposed to rabies and desperately needed immediate medical attention.

Even Dr. Denny Constantine, DVM, who carried out the studies thought that transmission of rabies to a human by a bat flying around in a room was essentially impossible. He tried to underscore the highly unusual conditions under which he had demonstrated aerial transmission—extended exposure (to 30 days) and the extreme saturation of the viruses in the cave room atmosphere.

Dr. Constantine also wrote: "Data available from the western United States do not support popular belief that an increase in bat rabies cases has occurred since the disease was first detected in the West in 1954."

Since the mid-1990s, Public Health officials have been publicizing in news releases and in reports to school officials the claim (especially to schoolteachers in the lower grades) that even touching a bat guarantees exposure to rabies. Some guidelines for persons carrying out lecture and demonstration sessions concerning bats require that all live bats be kept in airtight containers and students must not be allowed to touch a bat. Such procedures are to be followed even though the pet bat has been in captivity for months or years.

The panic over bat rabies as a threat to humans is an exaggerated, unwarranted reaction. Data still indicate that, while many species of bats may have been found to carry rabies, the incidence of actual cases is still very low. The number of human cases is much too small to warrant concern about an "outbreak."

RICKETTSIA ORGANISMS

*R*ickettsias are tiny organisms, between viruses and bacteria in size. Some recent classifications arrange them as a subgroup of bacteria. They, like viruses, are unable to reproduce outside of a cell in the host. Unlike viruses, they can be seen with a light microscope. Four types of diseases that affect humans are caused by rickettsias: Rocky Mountain spotted fever, rickettsial pox, typhus and ehrlichiosis.

Rocky Mountain Spotted Fever (Tick Fever)

Rocky Mountain spotted fever, sometimes called *tick fever,* is caused by the *Rickettsia rickettsii.* The disease was first discovered in 1899 in the Rocky Mountains, but most cases have been reported in the eastern United States and Canada. Several different rodents serve as reservoirs. The disease is not contagious except as transmitted by ticks of the family Ixodidae (usually a wood tick or dog tick) that have fed on an infected small mammal.

The number of reported human cases has varied recently from about 600 to 1,200 each year. Most cases are contracted between April and September.

Symptoms arise from 3 to 14 days after the tick bite, with eight days the average. Their onset is sudden and they include chills and fever (to 106F, 41C), severe headaches, and pain in the joints. In about 80 percent of the cases, a red rash develops about four days later, usually first on soles of the feet and palms of the hands, then spreading over the body. Untreated severe cases cause death in about two weeks.

Marmots (woodchucks), ground squirrels, chipmunks, flying squirrels, tree squirrels, deer mice, cotton rats, voles, Old World rats, and jumping mice are reservoirs.

Rickettsial Pox

This disease was first recognized in 1940. It is caused by a rickettsial organism, *Rickettsia akari,* that occurs in house mice and Old World rats. Mites that live on these rodents transmit the disease to humans.

The disease is usually mild. About eight days after being bitten by an infected mite, the person finds a red bump at the site of the bite. The bump enlarges, forms a blister, and then a scab. A few days later, a headache, fever (to 104F, 40C), chills, and muscle pains develop, followed with a rash that often covers the whole body.

The disease, even untreated, usually clears up in about one week.

This disease has been diagnosed in various parts of the United States, usually in larger cities, as well as in Russia.

Typhus

Four major forms of typhus are generally recognized: (1) epidemic, caused by *Rickettsia prowazekii* and transmitted from human to human by body lice; (2) Brill-Zinsser disease, a milder, recurring form of epidemic typhus; (3) scrub (or mite-borne) typhus, caused by *Rickettsia tsutsugamushi,* restricted mostly to eastern Asia, and transmitted from rodents to humans by larval mites (chiggers); and (4) murine typhus, caused by *Rickettsia mooseri* and transmitted from rodents to humans by fleas. It is this last variety that may affect humans in the United States and Canada.

Murine typhus was first described as a separate disease in 1931, although a mild typhuslike disease had been reported in the southeastern United States for about 30 years. Murine typhus is now known to occur in most parts of the United States and occasionally in Canada.

Symptoms in humans include chills and fever, aches and pains, severe headaches, and, after five days, a rash.

Although once found in the United States only in Old World rats in the Atlantic Coast cities, typhus is now known to occur in tree squirrels, ground squirrels, marmots, voles and other native rodents, as well as in opossums, rabbits and skunks. It only rarely occurs in pikas. Perhaps, as some speculate, the type of fleas that transmit the disease don't occur on pikas.

Ehrlichiosis

Ehrlichiosis is caused by *Ehrlichia chaffeensis,* a rickettsial organism that infects mainly white blood cells in the bloodstream. Other species in the genus *Ehrlichia* have been known for several years to infect horses and dogs.

Ehrlichiosis was first recognized as a human disease in 1987. Much is still to be learned about this disease, but ticks are thought to be the primary vector. Since its discovery, about 250 cases have been reported, mainly in the south-central and southeastern United States, especially in Georgia, Missouri, and Oklahoma. Most cases have developed in May, June or July.

Usually about seven days after a tick bite (but up to 21 days), the victim develops symptoms much like those seen in Rocky Mountain spotted fever. Chills and fever, headache, upset stomach and muscle aches are common. In about one case in five a rash develops. Severe complications, including kidney or respiratory failure, have occurred in some cases. A few fatalities have been recorded.

To date, no reservoir species has been discovered. However, based on patterns in other disease-causing rickettsia organisms, it's possible that one or more rodents serve as reservoirs.

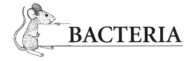

BACTERIA

*B*acteria (the singular is bacterium) are primitive, single-celled organisms. All are small and can only be seen with the aid of a microscope. They vary greatly in size, shape, and living requirements. Some thrive only in extreme conditions, such as in hot springs, sulphur springs, ocean depths, and even in the water of melting glaciers. No count of the number of species is yet possible but scientists estimate that half a million to three-quarters of a million different kinds of bacteria exist on earth today.

Most bacteria are free-living, but some can live only in the body of a host organism. Plants and animals alike serve as hosts for various bacterial infections. Humans are actual or potential hosts of several dozen different bacteria, some of which cause diseases. Six different bacterial diseases that involve rodents or rabbits as reservoir hosts are known to affect humans in the United States. Available antibiotics are usually effective if the diseases is diagnosed and treated promptly.

Relapsing Fevers (Tick Fever)

This disease—actually a conglomerate of closely related diseases—is caused by spirochetal bacteria of the genus *Borrelia*. Spirochetes are spiral-shaped bacteria. The bacteria that cause relapsing fevers infect birds and mammals in many parts of the world. Some species are transmitted from host to host by lice, others by ticks. The disease is sometimes referred to as "tick fever," a term that is also applied to Colorado tick fever (caused by a virus) and Rocky Mountain spotted fever (caused by a rickettsia organism).

Several variants of relapsing fever can be recognized. Most are caused by the bacteria living in the bloodstream and bodily tissues of the host. Another group, rarely seen in the United States, live in the human mouth.

One group of these spirochetes (some argue that they are only one, with minor regional differences) is transmitted from human to human by the human body louse (the plural is lice). These are known only in North Africa and India.

Another group (nine or more species, all in the genus *Borrelia*) are transmitted from a rodent reservoir to humans by ticks in the genus *Ornithodoros*. These species occur in Asia, Europe, Africa, North America, Central America and South America. Usually only one of the species occurs in a given region and each is transmitted by a different species of tick.

One species (*Borrelia burgdorfa*) causes the recently recognized Lyme disease, which is discussed later.

A bacterial organism that causes one type of relapsing fever in humans was first isolated and identified in Germany in 1868. Tick-borne relapsing fevers were first recognized in the United State in 1915. Most cases are contracted from exposures in rural or wilderness areas, mainly in the western United States and Canada. *Borrelia hermsii*, transmitted by *Ornithodoros hermsi*, is mainly found in forests above 3,000 feet in elevation but sometimes occurs at low elevations. *Borrelia turicatae*, transmitted by *Ornithodoros turica*, mainly occurs in semiarid grasslands. Rarely, *Borrelia mazzottii*, transmitted by *Ornithodoros talaje*, is found in semiarid areas. Some rare cases of *Borrelia parkeri*, transmitted by *Ornithodoros parkeri*, have been recorded.

Symptoms of relapsing fevers begin suddenly, four to 18 days after infection. They include chills and fever (to 105F, 40.6C), severe headaches, muscle aches, joint pains, coughing, and nausea. The symptoms persist for three to six days, disappear for seven to ten days, and recur in a milder form. Several relapses often occur and, even when the disease is untreated, recovery is usually complete. However, death has occurred in some cases, mainly in young children and elderly adults.

The actual number of cases of these relapsing fevers in humans is unknown, mainly because the disease is frequently not recognized and the symptoms are thought to be from some other cause.

Reservoir rodents include chipmunks, tree squirrels and voles.

Lyme Disease

Lyme disease is another bacterial, animal-borne illness that has received much publicity in recent years. The name is derived from Lyme, Connecticut, where the illness was first identified in 1975. In 1992, more than 9000 human cases were reported in the United States, mostly originating in May through August.

Cases have been reported in all of the 48 continental states, as well as in adjacent southern Canada. Most occur in the southeastern Canada, northeastern Atlantic coastal states, the upper Midwest, and northern California. The disease also occurs in Europe and Asia, where a slightly different variety of the bacterium is found.

This disease is caused by *Borrelia burgdorferi,* a bacterium transmitted to humans by the bite of ticks. Ticks become infected by feeding on diseased wild animals, including birds, deer, rabbits and rodents.

Symptoms of Lyme disease range from mild to drastic. Typically, redness of skin expands from the site of the bite, and often clears at the site and produces a large red ring. Smaller rings may appear on other parts of the body and last for days. Rash, aches and fever are common. Weeks after the symptoms disappear, some humans develop an irregular heartbeat, inflamed brain tissues and even paralyzed muscles of the face. Usually these symptoms disappear in a few days or weeks. Months later arthritis may develop.

Children appear to be more often exposed to this disease than adults, probably because they are most apt to encounter ticks that may be brought in by pet dogs.

The causative organism has also been found in chipmunks, deer mice, and wood rats.

Intestinal Bacterial Infections

The Enterobacteriaceae family of bacteria includes hundreds of varieties that are found throughout the world. By 1975, more than 1,600 sereotypes, or varieties, had been identified. These are often grouped into 11 genera. They occur in a wide variety of animals, including domestic and wild mammals as well as birds and even turtles. Apparently most of the bacteria are transmitted from animal to animal by contaminated food and water.

Some varieties of Enterobacteriaceae can cause intestinal infections in humans with fever and diarrhea as the most common symptoms. Because most of these infections don't last long and are usually mild, people often don't see a doctor, so most cases are never documented in health reports. One source estimates that probably 2-million cases occur in the United States each year, with only about 20,000 being reported.

"Food poisoning" and "bacillary dysentery" are well-known examples of intestinal bacterial infections. Most human infections are transmitted from human to human by contamination. To help avoid transmitting bacterial infections, obey those signs in restaurant bathrooms: "Wash your hands."

At least four genera within the family (*Salmonella, Shigella, Arizona,* and *Enchericha coli*) involve animals as reservoir hosts. These infectious bacteria can be transmitted from reservoir to humans by contaminated food or water or, more rarely, by direct contact or even by air. In most cases, humans have acquired these bacteria from chickens, eggs, livestock, cats, dogs, rabbits, lizards, turtles and even fish.

Salmonella has also been found in rodents. Laboratory and pet mice and rats, as well as wild species (including muskrats), are reservoirs. Most transmission has apparently been from contaminated food.

Leptospirosis (Weil's Syndrome)

This human disease is caused by the bacterium *Leptospira interrogans,* which occurs in various domestic and wild animals including rodents. It's transmitted to humans from the urine of infected animals through abraded skin or mucous membranes. This could happen if you actually touch something—a nest or remains of food or soil—that has bacteria on it, or if you consume water contaminated by the bacterium. The disease was first recognized in 1870 and the causative organism was determined in 1907.

Symptoms usually occur seven to 13 days after exposure. Onset is sudden. Victims suffer from chills and fever, severe muscular aches, headaches and redness of the eyes. These symptoms usually disappear after four to nine days, but after two to three days, they can recur along with a stiff neck. In some untreated cases, a severe form (Weil's syndrome) may develop, and it has caused some fatalities.

A number of different animals serve as reservoirs. Among domestic animals, dogs, cattle and swine are especially common. Among wild animals, fish, reptiles, amphibians, birds and various mammals have all been identified as reservoirs. Rodent reservoirs include house mice, Norway rats, black rats, deer mice, harvest mice, cotton rats, muskrats, marmots, voles, beavers and tree squirrels.

Plague

Plague, the disease, is caused by a bacterium, *Yersinia pestis* (formerly known as *Pasteurella pestis*) that is generally transmitted from rodents to humans by flea bites. People can also catch the disease by handling the flesh of a diseased animal, such as when skinning wild game. It's one of the most dangerous, and most frequently fatal, of the animal-borne diseases.

"Plague," the word, has been used for centuries to describe any scourge or calamity that is widespread and not easily remedied. Thus, a plague of locusts (grasshoppers) might destroy a crop, a plague of wolves might destroy a herd of sheep, or a plague of sickness might wipe out a village.

Human plague outbreaks have been associated with sick and dying rodents since biblical times. A series of pandemics (widespread epidemics) has been documented over the centuries. Perhaps the most notable was the Great Pestilence, later known as the Black Death, that is reputed to have caused as many as 25-million deaths in Europe in the Middle Ages.

Yersinia pestis was identified in 1894 as the bacterium that causes plague. When it was isolated in both dead humans and dead rats, scientists thought that rats served as the main animal host for the disease. In 1896 the role of rat fleas in the transmission of the disease was determined, and two years later, plague in wild rodents was confirmed. These discoveries were made in Hong Kong, Formosa (Taiwan), and India. Laboratory tests have shown that even a single bacterium can cause a major infection in an animal.

Three different forms of plague are recognized in humans: bubonic, septicemic and pneumonic, all caused by the same bacterium. Incubation usually lasts from a few hours to a few days, but some cases involved longer times.

Bubonic plague generally involves the rapid onset of chills and fever, headache, and extreme fatigue. The most characteristic symptom is the development of a bubo in the groin or armpit region. A bubo is an enlargement of a lymphatic gland, along with an extremely painful swelling of the surrounding area. Often a sore develops at the site of the flea bite.

Septicemic plague, which occurs when the bacteria invade the bloodstream, is usually a secondary stage of bubonic plague in which no bubo is formed. Some infected people have a bloody rash. High fevers often don't develop, as they do in the bubonic variety.

In pneumonic plague, the bacteria settle primarily in the lungs, rather than in a bubo or in the bloodstream. In this form, the bacteria can be transmitted directly from human to human by breathing.

When untreated, about 60 percent of those with bubonic plague die. In septicemic and pneumonic plague, the odds are even worse: approaching 100 percent. In these two forms, death usually occurs after a sickness of only one to three days.

Plague is generally a disease of rodents, with over 200 species known to be carriers. Depending on the types of rodents involved, plague is often classified as either "urban" or "sylvatic."

Urban plague is carried by rodent species that live in close association with humans. In the New World, these are mainly house mice, black rats, and Norway rats—all introduced from the Old World into North America. In most of the United States, rodent-control programs have kept the populations of these animals low. As a result, no cases of urban plague have been reported for a number of years.

Sylvatic plague involves rodent species that live in rural areas. Today plague is persistent in wild rodents in the southern United States, South America, Africa, and Central Asia. Plague has been found in marmots, ground squirrels, chipmunks, prairie dogs, tree squirrels, deer mice, wood rats and voles.

Tularemia (Rabbit Fever)

This disease, caused by the bacterium *Francisella tularensis* which occurs mainly in rodents and rabbits, is transmitted to humans when they're bitten by flies, fleas, ticks or lice. It can also be contracted by contact with the flesh or blood of infected animals. About half of the human cases are the result of tick bites. The number of reported human cases varies from year to year, usually ranging from 150 to 300.

The causative bacterium was first isolated in the early 1900s from rodents in Tulare County, California—hence the name "tularemia."

Symptoms can occur in three days; rare cases have taken as long as 108 days to develop after exposure. Symptoms, which appear suddenly, include chills and fever (to 104F, 40C), severe headaches, muscle aches, joint pains, often nausea, and often extreme fatigue. If the bacteria enter the body through the skin, a sore appears at the entrance site.

Tularemia is called *rabbit fever* because rabbits are often infected. Humans often get infected while they prepare rabbits or other game for food. Among rodents, tularemia has been detected in marmots, ground squirrels, tree squirrels, beavers, voles, muskrats, Old World rats, house mice and porcupines. It occurs in various other mammals, both wild and domestic.

PARASITIC DISEASES

A parasite is an organism that lives in or on another organism. It depends on the host organism for its food and life support. Without the host, it can't survive. Two types of parasites, protozoa and fungi, cause diseases that can affect humans.

Protozoa are usually single-celled organisms but they're larger than bacteria. One of them is a protozoan. They're often classified as primitive members of the animal kingdom. Though some protozoa are parasitic, living in higher animals, most are free-living, usually existing in water. Protozoa can cause babesiosis, Chagas' disease, and giardiasis in humans.

A fungus is a primitive plant, without chlorophyll. Mushrooms, mildews, smuts, and molds are all members of this group, and all are parasites. The human diseases that are carried by fungi include coccidiomycosis and histoplasmosis.

PROTOZOA-CAUSED DISEASES

Babesiosis

This disease is caused by a parasitic protozoan, *Babesia microti*, that infests red blood cells of various animals. Rodents have been proved to be reservoirs, and the same kinds of ticks involved in the transmission of Lyme disease are the major vectors. Another species of this protozoan causes Texas fever (also called *cattle tick fever*) in cattle.

Since babesiosis was first recognized in the United States in 1968, more than 450 cases have been reported. Most cases occur in summer, and have been caused by exposure to ticks in the Northeast, especially on coastal islands. Similar cases have been reported in California, Washington and Wisconsin, though researchers aren't yet sure this is the same disease.

Symptoms are very similar to those of malaria: tiredness and fatigue about seven days after exposure, followed by chills, fever, headache and muscle soreness. Most cases are mild but some lead to anemia and kidney failure. Some cases have been fatal, especially in older patients. Drugs used in the treatment of malaria have been used with limited success.

Reservoirs include deer mice and voles.

Chagas' Disease

This disease is caused by a protozoan, *Trypanosoma cruzi,* that is most common in Central and South America. Current estimates are that several-million people in those regions are affected. Brazil is especially heavily infected.

Most cases occur in people who live in marginal housing that is infested with kissing bugs (also called the "cone-nosed bug"—family Reduviidae, subfamily Triatominae, genus *Triatoma*). These blood-feeding insects transmit the parasite from reservoir animals (including opossums and armadillos) and infected humans (usually of the same family) to the new host.

The disease occurs when a bug, feeding on an infected mammal, passes the protozoan through its intestine and leaves its waste on the skin of a human. The human then unknowingly scratches the insect bite area, contaminating the wound (or often the eyes) by rubbing the waste into the break in the skin. The name, Chagas' disease, comes from the Brazilian physician Carlos Chagas, who identified the tropical disease in 1912.

The first symptoms of Chagas' disease are often a small red sore on the skin or swollen, red, inflamed eyes. Weeks later, the sore appears to heal and the crusty scab is lost, leaving a small, dark scar. In some cases, this may be followed by fevers, swelling of the lymph glands, and body and skin rashes. In severe cases the heart is affected and the victims experience chest pains and shortness of breath. When the nervous system is involved, the patient has convulsions. Some cases are fatal.

In the United States, Chagas' disease occurs occasionally in the southern and southwestern states. There spiny pocket mice, cotton rats and wood rats are reservoirs.

Giardiasis (Beaver Fever)

This is the most common human parasitic disease in the United States and especially in western Canada. Caused by a parasitic protozoan, *Giardia lamblia,* it infests the inner surface of the human gut, especially the small intestine. The result is an infectious diarrhea. In daycare centers it has occurred in 2 of 10,000 children.

Contaminated food and water are the usual sources of infestation. Childcare centers and nursing homes are especially subject to outbreaks of giardiasis if strict sanitary controls are not maintained. In most cases, cysts of the protozoan enter the person's digestive tract through food or water that contains fecal wastes of humans of animals.

In humans infected with giardiasis, chronic diarrhea begins about three weeks after infection. They also experience nausea and other abdominal discomfort. Prolonged infections may produce weight loss as a result of poor absorption of digested food in the intestine. Some cases show spontaneous recovery but in others, the human remains infected for years.

In rural areas surface water supplies are sometimes infested with *Giardia cysts.* Some of this contamination probably comes from human fecal wastes, but native rodents have also been found to serve as sources of contamination. For a number of years, beavers were thought to be a major reservoir of this protozoan in the wilderness. Recent studies indicate that cattle and sheep may be the major reservoir; beavers, like humans, are probably a secondary host.

The causative parasite has been found in beavers, voles, muskrats and kangaroo rats.

FUNGI-CAUSED DISEASES

Coccidiomycosis (Valley Fever)

Coccidiomycosis is an infection transmitted by a fungus, *Coccidioides immitis* of the family Endomycotales. In nature the fungus grows on decaying vegetation in the soil. It is especially common in arid and semiarid regions of the Southwest, where the first human case was diagnosed in 1896 in the San Joaquin Valley, California. Thus, the familiar name, "valley fever."

Exposure usually occurs when a person inhales spores of the fungus. The incubation period varies from a week to a month, with recognizable symptoms being observable in 10 to 16 days.

The fungus infects human lungs, and initial symptoms may include chills and fever, headaches, coughs, sore throat and aches and pains, especially in the back. Allergic reactions may also occur and some patients develop a rash. As the disease spreads to other parts of the body, a wide variety of symptoms can occur. They're usually associated with the parts of the body being infected. Infection is usually mild, and people recover even from untreated cases. In only rare cases, it's fatal.

The coccidiomycosis fungus lives in the soil and, strictly speaking, doesn't depend upon an animal reservoir for its existence. However, during dry seasons, a few of the fungi have been isolated on surface soils, and high populations exist in the soils in and around underground rodent burrows. In some regions, increased numbers of cases have been documented in newly developed subdivisions where the soils (and the rodent burrows) have been disturbed and windblown dust is common.

Histoplasmosis

Histoplasmosis is an infection caused by a different fungus, *Histoplasma capsulatum*. Like valley fever, the disease is acquired by breathing the spores of the fungus. It's widely distributed and common in much of the midwestern United States and adjacent parts of Canada. Most cases are never diagnosed, but are thought to have been a severe cold. Up to half of the people who have spent most of their first 21 years of life in the Midwest show a positive skin test for the disease.

Some cases are much more severe and a few are fatal. In these cases the fungi become established in the body, often growing in the lung cavity. In rare cases, the disease simulates other illnesses, including septic fever and anemia. It can also involve the lymph nodes and cause tuberculosislike symptoms in the lungs and chest.

The fungus grows on decaying vegetation, especially in and around barnyards and other areas where animal and bird manures enrich the soil. In recent years some serious cases of histoplasmosis have been associated with exposure to the spores in damp caves and caverns where the fungus apparently thrives on bat guano (manure). The fungus has been detected in some damp caves in central Arizona. The most severe cases have resulted from infections contracted in bat caves in Mexico, with the sickness developing after the victim returned to the United States or Canada.

CHRONIC FATIGUE SYNDROME

Chronic Fatigue Syndrome (CFS), sometimes called the *Epstein-Barr Syndrome,* is not, strictly speaking, a disease, but rather is a list of symptoms. Symptoms include severe fatigue that results in reduced physical abilities for periods of six months or more: Extremely weak muscles, reduced mental abilities (loss of memory), fever, sore throat and joints, and the inability to do any sustained exercise. The cause? As is usual with syndromes, there is no one cause. However, some cases appear to have been caused by Lyme Disease or Tick Fever.

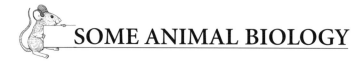 SOME ANIMAL BIOLOGY

As we have already seen, these diseases all involve some rodent, bat or rabbit as a host from which the causative organism (virus, rickettsia organism, bacterium or parasite) makes it way, by way of some vector, to a human. In this primer we are mainly concerned only with bats, rabbits and hares, and rodents, because they are the major reservoirs of animal diseases that affect humans.

This chapter outlines of some of the major natural factors that influence the numbers and distribution of these potential disease reservoirs. Because bats, rodents and rabbits are all animals, it is no surprise that most of these natural factors control the lives of all animals.

For the novice, we start this section with a quick review of the biologist's system of applying names to the different kinds of animals and of arranging closely related kinds in groups: CLASSIFICATION.

The number of actual or potential reservoirs (individual bats, rodents or rabbits) in an area certainly influences the likelihood of a disease being transmitted to a human. More reservoirs equals greater chance of exposure! For this reason, a general discussion of factors influencing population size is included: POPULATIONS.

Because the natural conditions in the wild are varied, it is not surprising that not all kinds of mammals occur everywhere. Tree-dwelling squirrels don't survive long in a large grassland. Beavers are not found in the middle of deserts. A general knowledge of the special life requirements of the various kinds of bats, rodents and rabbits helps one understand their numbers and distribution. This helps you evaluate your degree of potential exposure and helps identify any individuals seen. Some of these factors are summarized in the section: ECOLOGY.

Finally, when populations of a potential vector are high and a disease is known to be present, control measures are often necessary. Some techniques are outlined in the section: POPULATION CONTROL.

Classification

The following general survey of animal classification (arranging the various kinds in meaningful groups) apply equally well to all animals.

Animals are the members of the Animal Kingdom. This Kingdom include the single-celled protozoans (amoeba), the Invertebrates (animals without a backbone such as sponges, worms, and insects) and the Vertebrates (animals with a backbone, the fish, amphibians, reptiles, birds and mammals).

Mammals, with which were are primarily concerned here, are vertebrate animals that have fur, warm blood and give birth to live young. Based on differences in structure and habits, zoologists generally recognize 17 different major groups (orders) of living mammals, as well as several extinct orders.

Here we are concerned with only three orders of mammals— Chiroptera containing the bats, Lagomorpha containing the hares and rabbits, and Rodentia—the Rodents.

The bats (Chiroptera) are the only mammals with true flight. The forearm and digits (fingers) are modified to support a soft, thin structure of skin—the flight membrane. Size is generally small, the largest in North America being the Mastiff Bat, with a wingspread of about 21 inches and a weight of just over two ounces. Food consists mainly of night-flying insects, although several feed on fruit or nectar. A few in tropical regions feed on larger animals including frogs, fish and even other bats. Two kinds feed on blood (vampires).

The hares and rabbits (Lagomorpha) are modified for feeding on low vegetation, generally in open grasslands. The tail is reduced, the pinna (ears) are elongated (detecting at a distance any approaching enemy), and the hind-limbs are enlarged (for leaping and fast running). The teeth are modified for feeding on vegetation. The front teeth are reduced to four above (two large incisors with a tiny tooth behind each) and two incisors below. The cheek-teeth (molars and premolars) are modified for cutting and grinding of plant leaves and stems. Weights range from 4.5 ounces (125 grams) to 5.7 pounds (2.5 kilograms).

The rodents (Rodentia) are by far and away the most diverse and most numerous mammals, making up almost 44% of the living species of mammals. They range in size from the tiny Pygmy Mouse (about 4 inches [100 mm] in total length and weighing 0.4 ounce [10 grams]) to the giant South American Capybara (with a total length of about 4 feet (1300mm) and a weight of up to 250 pounds [113 kilograms]). All have the teeth reduced to two incisors above and two below and no molars.

Several kinds (species) occur in each of the three orders considered here (Chiroptera—bats; Lagomorpha—hares and rabbits; Rodentia—rodents). Based upon the relationships among the different members of each order, the various kinds are grouped in Families, such as the Squirrel Family (Sciuridae) and the Beaver Family (Castoridae) in the Order Rodentia.

Zoologists are still discovering new kinds of animals, especially among the insects, nematode worms, and the mites and chiggers. Each species is assigned a scientific name, consisting of a Latin or Latinized noun—the genus—and a Latin or Latinized adjective—the species. For example, the scientific name of the cow is *Bos taurus*. It is based upon the Latin noun, "bos" meaning cow and an adjective form of the Greek word, "taurus," meaning steer. The noun (genus) is always capitalized; the specific name is not. Botanists, however, retain the capital in the specific name when it is based on a proper name (person or place). Being Latin, a scientific name remains the same, no matter what language or even alphabet is in the accompanying text.

Common names are simply the name applied to the animal by most people. Obviously many species are often grouped under a single common name. For example, "gopher." The University of Minnesota "Golden Gophers," a football team, is based on a ground squirrel in the area. In the western United

States, a "gopher" is a member of the pocket gopher family, Geomyidae, while in Florida a "gopher" is a land tortoise that digs a hole in the ground. In contrast, about 50 years ago a zoologist tried to compiled a list of all the different common names that had been applied to the English or House Sparrow (*Passer domesticus*) in the various parts of the world. His list included more than 30 different "common names."

The scientific names and common names used here are, in general, as in the *Checklist of Vertebrates of the United States, the U. S. Territories, and Canada* (Resource Publication 166 of the U. S. Dept. of Interior Fish and Wildlife Service).

Populations

In general terms, the size of a population can be expressed by the formula P = BP - ER [P (number of individuals) equals BP (=biotic potential) minus ER (environmental resistance)].

Biotic Potential is the rate at which the number of individual can increase under ideal conditions (unlimited food, water, living space, no enemies, no diseases, no old age . . .).

Environmental Resistance is the total of all factors that prevent reproduction (starvation, temperatures, crowding, diseases, parasites, enemies, death . . .).

The BP (Biotic Potential) of mammals (as well as all other living organisms) is much greater than the numbers that can exist in nature. However, the biotic potential varies greatly among the various species being considered here.

Most bats only have a single young each year. In the kinds that occur in Canada and the United States the young is born in the late spring after a gestation period of several weeks. For most, the average life expectancy is probably 6-8 years for females and 8-9 years for males but some banded individuals have been recovered after 30 years. Obviously, even under ideal conditions, several years are necessary for population to recover from any massive destruction caused by diseases or humans.

Compared to bats and the larger mammals, rabbits and most rodents reach reproductive age in a short time and have a short gestation period, a large number of young in a litter—and a short life span. Cottontail rabbits can have three or four litters each year with up to nine young in each litter.

Most rodents, especially most rats and mice, have spectacular reproductive rates. The House mouse is sexually mature at the age of 35 days and a female's first litter (up to 12 or more in number) can be born about 19 days later. In captivity, one female may have six litters in one year. One of the Voles has a gestation period of 21 days and has six to eight young per litter. One female, in captivity, gave birth to 17 litters in one year and a second female gave birth to 13 litters before she was one year old. If we assume: one adult pair, that all young produced will live, and that the sex ratio of the young is one to one, then, using the above figures, in one year more than 1,000,000 individuals could result from one pair.

In contrast, tree squirrels, marmots, prairie dogs and muskrats do not breed until they are one year old. Beavers reach maturity in the second year and porcupines breed in their third year.

Average life expectancy of most rats and mice is just a few weeks, especially in nature. Even in captivity few live beyond a second year. Marmots and Tree squirrels rarely survive more than one year in nature (up to 15 years in captivity), and Beavers and Porcupines, four to five years (up to 20 years in captivity).

In nature, the ER (environmental resistance) takes its toll. As a result, fluctuations in population size are normal. In most rodents and rabbits the biotic potential, in "good times" (improved food, weather, etc.) can have large populations develop in a few weeks or months. These high populations often result in food shortages, diseases and population crashes. Total populations are usually smallest at the beginning of a breeding season and largest just at the end of the season. In the short-lived rats and mice, these periods are in the spring and in the early fall.

Biologists concerned with the actual or potential effect of populations on such things as crop and pasture production, reforestation projects, and potential for disease outbreaks often attempt to determine the populations of various mammals.

Because no birth certificates, census records or social security numbers are available, biologists make "educated guesses" as to numbers. Considered in these estimates is knowledge of the habits of the species being studied.

Daily and seasonal variations in time of activity can greatly influence estimates of population size. Some species are usually active only during the day (crepuscular) while others are active at night (nocturnal). Weather conditions influence activity, with many seeking shelter during adverse conditions (rain, storms, heat and cold). Even the brightness of moonlight affects the activity of nocturnal mammals, especially those that live in open areas such as grasslands and deserts.

Seasonal differences in activity must also be considered. Some rodents and many bats spend much of the cold season in hibernation. Some bats migrate southward. Some species that spend the summer in Canada move south for the winter— some kinds even moving to Mexico. Most Ground squirrels and Tree squirrels, during hot, dry periods, are most active either early or late in the day and many of the native mice are not as active during the hottest summer months as they are in the cooler months.

All of these factors, and others, are taken into account in a biologist's "educated guess" of population size. If estimates involve trapping, marking, releasing and retrapping, the effect of seasonal variations in reactions to a bait must be considered.

Multi-annual fluctuations in population size are common. Weather conditions resulting in increased plant growth (food production) in some years are generally followed by increases in rodent populations. However, conditions favorable to one species may not be favorable to others. For example, unusually good rains in the winter and spring result in the fabled "desert bloom" in the southwestern deserts. This results in the production of many seeds of the annual plants. This favors the rapid in populations of the seed-eating Pocket mice and Kangaroo rats but has little effect on the populations of Wood rats and Ground squirrels. Conversely, a rain cycle that results in greatly increased growth of cacti and various perennial shrubs has little effect on Pocket mice and Kangaroo rat populations but causes increases in the populations of Ground squirrels and Wood rats.

Some spectacular "rabbit plagues" have occurred in the Great Plains areas, usually after a mild winter followed by a dry spring. These conditions result in a high survival rate of the newborn young.

Ecology

Useful in determining the kinds of bats, rodents and rabbits are present in a given area is some knowledge of the habitat preferences of each. Factors defining the habitat of a given species include latitude and/or elevation, vegetation, climate, soil type, and even place of activity (underground tunnels, in trees, in the air . . .).

In the northern latitudes of Alaska and Canada, no bats and relatively few kinds of rodents and rabbits are present. Similar conditions exist at high elevations in mountains even in the southwestern United States. In general, the farther south you go, the more kinds of bats are present. Three species are known from southern Alaska, one as a summer resident. Canada has 15 species, three of which migrate southward for the winter. Maine has eight species, three of which migrate southward. In contrast, 30 different species have been recorded from Arizona and 86 in the Central American country of Costa Rica.

The type of dominant vegetation of a region greatly influences the kinds and numbers of mammals present. The tundra in the far north and similar vegetation types above timberline on high mountains, evergreen forests, deciduous forests, brush zones, grasslands, deserts, marshes and aquatic plants in water are some major types. Each of these areas has one or more characteristic kinds of rodents. Examples are flying squirrels in forests, prairie dogs in grasslands and muskrats feeding on aquatic vegetation.

Others feed mainly underground (pocket gophers), in trees (flying squirrels), in the air (bats) or in or near water (muskrats).

Even when an individual is in a favorable habitat, it does not wander around at random through the countryside. Rather, each lives most of its live in a very limited area termed its *home range.* The special ways of life each influences the size of the home range. A fossorial (burrowing) Pocket gopher has a smaller home range than does a Ground squirrel of similar size.

Bats, with their ability to fly for long distances, have much larger home ranges but also spend most of their time in a specific feeding or roosting area.

Size also influences home-range size. Tiny mice have a tiny home range while a hare may routinely cover several acres in its search for food. The part of the home range that is defended from others of the same species is termed a *territory.* Some rodents are highly territorial and quite solitary in their behavior. Others, especially some of the Ground squirrels and Prairie dogs, are extremely social and live in colonies that have social structure.

Several species have modifications of the body that make life easier (or even possible) in some of these special habitats. Examples include the wings of bats; the gliding membranes of the flying squirrel; the scaled, flattened tail and webbed feet of the beaver and muskrat; and the long hind legs of Jack rabbits. Such specializations are in the accounts of the various kinds of mammals that make up the next section.

As indicated, even the time of activity differs from species to species. Bats feed at night and spend the day in dark shelters. Rabbits and rodents spend part of each day resting and sleeping. Some are nocturnal, others are diurnal and especially in hot and cold periods, some of each group become crepuscular, with most activity at dusk or dawn.

Most bats feed on flying insects and some rodents (jumping mice, marmots, the ground hog and some ground squirrels) feed on green vegetation, neither of which are available in the cold season. Some bats migrate to warm regions in the south but most, like the green vegetation feeding rodents, become fat and sleep (hibernate) in some protected, cool place during cold weather. In extreme cases, some marmots and ground squirrels in northern areas hibernate for more than six months each year.

Most of the pocket mice combine hibernation (surviving on stored fat) with the storage of seeds in underground caches (for winter meals) as a means of surviving periods of low temperatures and little food.

Population Control

Natural—At times the numbers of rodents or rabbits exceed the "carrying capacity" of their habitat. In other words, the amount of available food, water, or other necessary item does not provide the needs of all members of the population. At such times some individuals become weak and are subject to diseases, parasites, and increased probability of being captured by a predator. The population is soon reduced to the level that can be supported in the region. In extreme situations, almost the entire population dies.

Little is known about the population dynamics in most bats. Some large-scale die-offs have been recorded and have been attributed to poisoning by insecticides or by some unspecified disease.

Human efforts—When rabbits, rodents or bats become too numerous, or invade man's buildings, some sort of control may become necessary. Obviously, some knowledge of the animal's habits becomes useful in such attempts. Most native rabbits and rodents rarely, if ever, enter buildings. In fact, many kinds do not survive in cultivated areas. At times, some species feed in gardens, yards, and cultivated fields but maintain their dens in adjacent, relatively natural habitats such as fence rows.

Native rodents that do routinely move into areas of human disturbance (buildings) include Wood rats (=Pack rats) and Deer mice, Tree and Flying squirrels (attics of buildings), Pocket gophers (golf courses, fields of root-crops—especially alfalfa), and Voles (pastures, hayfields and other grassy areas).

The Old World mouse and rats are usually the rodents that are present in buildings and in the areas disturbed by man's agricultural activities. Over the years these rodents have learned that the stored grains and other foodstuffs of man are an excellent source of food. They have learned to travel with man (in boats, trucks, etc.) and have accompanied him throughout the world. They are termed *commensals* of man. The House Mice that live away from buildings are almost always found in abandoned cultivated fields and overgrazed pastures. In the cold season, they often move back into buildings.

Two general methods of controlling bat, rodent and rabbit populations are available to humans: habitat manipulation and extermination.

One type of habitat manipulation is bat or rodent proofing—probably in many cases the most cost-effective long-term control. Screening or sealing of places of entry into buildings is usually a permanent deterrent.

If you just remove an unwanted bat or rodent, the vacant "niche" will probably be attractive to another looking for a place to live. For example, at a home in the foothills just at the edge of one southwestern city, a Wood rat (Pack rat) moved in from the surrounding native vegetation and built its den under a deck. The homeowner live-trapped it and moved it some miles away. That year a bountiful food supplies caused a large increase in Pack rat populations. The surplus young were all trying to find places to live. During the following two or three months, 18 different rats found the same place to live. Each was trapped and moved away. Rodent-proofing would have been useful!

Another habitat manipulation involves the use of *repellents.* Unfortunately, repellents rarely work very well in bat, rabbit or rodent control. In many cases, especially in open areas, the cost of a useful amount of repellant is prohibitive. When used in buildings, the amount needed to be effective is often sufficient to be a human repellant! Devices that plug into a wall socket and generate some "repellant wave" appear to be generally useless. How can such devices live up to the advertised claims of "repelling all unwanted rats, mice, bugs and birds," but do not affect household pets?

Extermination can be one of several methods including live-trapping and removal, kill trapping, poison baits and poison gasses. All require knowledge, supplies and equipment. Probably in most cases (especially the use of poisons) these should be carried out by a professional pest-control contractor.

Trapping generally involves the use of baits but sometimes unbaited traps can be successfully set in runways or trails. Various types of traps are available. Most are designed for rather specific usage: live traps, mouse traps, rat traps, gopher traps, squirrel traps, beaver traps . . . The selection of a proper trap is a must. Obviously, most squirrel traps are equipped with trigger mechanisms that a mouse could not set off. The operating mechanisms vary from guillotines to snares and spring traps, each of which require different techniques of operation.

Bait selection is just as important as trap selection. The classical "cheese" works with some House mice but is almost a repellant to all but the hungriest of some other species. A mixture of rolled oats and peanut butter is an acceptable bait to many rodents. Various studies of bait acceptance have shown that a given bait may be attractive to a species at one season of the year but not at other seasons. A study of Voles showed that green grass was an attractive bait in the winter but was refused in the summer. At that time, small containers of water were preferred. Smorgasbord experiments involving fruits, grains, seeds, rolled oats, peanut butter and others, may be necessary to find the favored bait for your troublesome rodent.

Poisons involve all of the problems of successful baiting (to get the poison into the rodent) plus all of the potential dangers to humans (children, adults), pets, and domestic animals. Further, many rodents soon learn to recognize the poison (odor? taste? ESP?). In the United States, most poisons are strictly controlled by the EPA (Environmental Protection Agency). Even the professional exterminators are limited in what they can use.

Poison gasses? Wow! Now we are talking about some serious killing techniques. Next we will be talking about Napalm! Carbon monoxide from the exhaust of a gasoline engine can sometimes be piped into a rodent's burrow. Of course, without proper care, carbon monoxide can eliminate the controller (SUICIDE), a child or some other human (MURDER ONE?), or other living creatures in the area.

IF POISON USAGE IS NECESSARY, YOU SHOULD SEEK PROFESSIONAL HELP.

Main Bats, Rodents and Rabbits in the United States and Canada

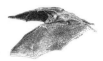

The arrangement of families and subfamilies used here is the one used in Wilson and Reeder, *Mammal Species of the World*, second edition, published by the Smithsonian Institution Press in association with the American Society of Mammalogists (see references section). The number of genera and species follows, in general, the *Checklist of Vertebrates of the United States, the U.S. Territories, and Canada*, Resource Publication 166 of the U.S. Department of the Interior, Fish and Wildlife Service.

In past times scientists grouped the rabbits and the rodents into a single order of mammals, termed *Glires*. However, most publications in recent decades place the rabbits and their relatives in the Order Lagomorpha and the rodents in the Order Rodentia. The major types of bats, rodents, and rabbits, in the United States and Canada, are listed in Table 4. Because no native rabbits or rodents and only one bat occur in Hawaii, distribution in this state is not given.

Table 4
Major Types of Bats, Rodents, and Lagomorphs in the United States and Canada

Note: "Resident bats" usually make only a minor shift from the summer roost to the winter hibernal habitat. They may travel up to a hundred miles to a suitable cave. "Migrating bats" may move hundreds (or even thousands) of miles.

Major Type (Number of Species)	Weight	Activity
Bats (41 species)		
Ghost-Faced Bat Family (1 species)		
Ghost bat (1)	0.5 oz.	resident

Table 4 *continued*

Major Type (Number of Species)	Weight	Activity
New World Leaf-Nosed Bat Family (5 species)		
Short-eared nectar feeders (3)	0.6 oz.	migrating
Big-eared insect feeders (2)	0.3-0.4 oz.	resident
Plain-Nosed Bat Family (29 species)		
Mouse-eared bats (14)	0.2-0.4 oz.	resident
Big brown bat (1)	0.6 oz.	resident
Pipistrelles (2)	0.1-0.3 oz.	resident
Evening bat (1)	0.4 oz.	resident
Tree bats		
Silver-haired bat (1)	0.4 oz.	migrating
Hoary bat (1)	1 oz.	migrating
Red bats (2)	0.4 oz.	migrating
Yellow bats (2)	0.5 oz.	resident
Big-eared bats (2)	0.4 oz.	resident
Spotted bat (1)	0.6 oz.	resident
Allen's big-eared bat (1)	0.45 oz.	resident
Pallid bat (1)	0.7 oz.	resident
Free-Tailed Bat Family (6 species)		
Brazilian free-tailed (1)	0.4 oz.	migrating
Large free-tailed (2)	0.5-0.9 oz.	resident
Mastiff bats (3)	1.2-1.6 oz.	resident
Rodents (199 species)		
Mountain Beaver Family (1 species)		
Mountain beaver (1)	2 lb.	Underground, mainly at night, all year

Table 4 *continued*

Major Type (Number of Species)	Weight	Activity
Squirrel Family (62 species)		
Flying squirrels (2)	6 oz.	In trees, at night, all year
Marmots (5)	to 20 lb.	At day during summer, hiernate in winter
Prairie dogs (4)	2 lb.	At day during summer, hiernate in winter
Ground squirrels (17)	4 oz. to 2 lb.	At day during summer, hiernate in winter
Antelope squirrels (4)	4 oz.	At day during summer, hiernate in cold winter
Chipmunks (22)	2 oz.	At day, hibernate in coldest weather
Red squirrels (2)	8 oz.	At day, ground and trees, all year
Tree squirrels (6)	1 lb.	At day, ground and trees, all year
North American Burrowing Rodent Family (13 species)		
Pocket gophers (13)	6-10 oz.	Day or night, underground, all year
Beaver Family (1 species)		
Beaver (1)	to 60 lb.	In or near water, all year

Table 4 *continued*

Major Type (Number of Species)	Weight	Activity
North American Desert Rodent Family (36 species)		
Kangaroo mice (2)	0.5 oz.	At night, all but coldest weather
Spiny pocket mice (9)	0.5-1 oz.	At night, hibernate in cold weather
Silky pocket mice (9)	0.2-0.8 oz.	At night, hibernate fall to spring
Kangaroo rats (16)	1.3-3.2 oz.	At night, all year
Rats and Mice Family (76 species)		
Rice rat (1)	2.6 oz.	Mostly at night, all year
Harvest mice (5)	0.5-0.7 oz.	Mostly at night, all year
Pygmy mouse (1)	0.4 oz.	At night, all year
Deer mice (17)	0.8-1.5 oz.	At night, all year
Grasshopper mice (2)	1.2 oz.	At night, all year
Cotton rats (4)	to 3.5 oz.	Day and night, all year
Wood rats (8)	6-11 oz.	At night, all year
Voles and meadow mice (31)	1-3.5 oz.	Day and night, all year
Muskrats (2)	4 lb	In or near water, at night, all year
House mouse (1)	0.7 oz.	Mainly at night in human habitats
Old World rats (2) (Norway and black)	10 oz.	Mainly at night in human habitats
Jumping Mice and Rats Family (4 species)		
Jumping mice (4)	0.8 oz.	At night, hibernate in cold weather

Table 4 *continued*

Major Type (Number of Species)	Weight	Activity
Porcupine Family (1 species)		
Porcupine (1)	18 lb.	Mainly at night in forests or brush
Lagomorphs (16 species)		
Pika Family (2 species)		
Pikas (2)	5-7 oz.	At day, all year
Hares and Rabbits Family (14 species)		
Hares and jackrabbits (6)	2-9 lb.	Mostly night, all year
Cottontails (8)	1-6 lb.	Mostly night, all year

BATS (Order Chiroptera)

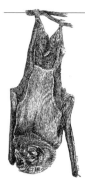

Bats are second only to rodents in diversity of living species. Currently 925 living species (177 genera, 17 families) are known around the world. In Canada and the United States, only 41 species, grouped in 19 genera and 4 families, are generally recognized.

For our purposes, these 41 species are grouped into 18 different "major types." For example, all 14 species in the genus *Myotis* are classified as "mouse-eared bats." While a mouse-eared bat can be rather easily identified from the features indicated here, even professional mammalogists sometimes have difficulties distinguishing among the 14 species.

Measurements given reflect an average value. Just as humans do, wild animals vary in size and weight, depending on differences in age, gender, health, and even season of the year. Most bats become much heavier (from stored fat) in the fall before the beginning of a migration trek or a winter of hibernation. Some vary as much as 40 percent.

Probably most useful for identification purposes is the length of the forearm.

The 4 families of bats in the United States are:

Ghost-Faced Bat Family
(Mormoopidae—1 species, 1 major type)

New World Leaf-Nosed Bat Family
(Phyllostomidae—5 species, 2 major types)

Plain-Nosed Bat Family
(Vespertilionidae—29 species, 12 major types)

Free-Tailed Bat Family
(Molossidae—6 species, 3 major types)

In 1954 rabies was recognized in insectivorous bats in the United States. Since then, it has been found in bats in Canada. At some time one or more species in each family has tested positive for rabies. Three groups are most commonly found to be infected:

1. Tree bats. Bats of this species spend their days roosting in the open or hiding in clumps of leaves on the bark of trees. They make long north-south migrations each year, some from Canada to the southern United States, others going even farther south into Mexico. Especially while migrating, they often hang up for a day in a place that can be detected by humans and their pet cats and dogs.

2. Cave bats. These are often found in the summer in the cracks, crevices, attics and belfries of various buildings. Because their day roosts are in cities and towns, as well as in remote forests and mountains, they are commonly encountered by humans and their pet cats and dogs.

3. The Brazilian free-tailed bats (also called *Mexican free-tailed* and *guano bat*). These are inhabitants of the southern parts of the United States, and millions of them often congregate in summer maternity colonies. The famous bat flight from Carlsbad Caverns National Park in New Mexico is made up of this species. Even larger colonies are known to live in west-central Texas.

Many of these bats spend the summer in an area from western Oklahoma and central Texas westward to southeastern California, and move southward into Mexico for the winter season. During both their southward and northward movements, they often spend a few days or weeks roosting at nights in attics, cracks, and crevices of buildings or in crevices in highway and railroad bridges. These bats too are often detected by humans and their pets.

GHOST-FACED BAT FAMILY
(Mormoopidae)

Members of this family (8 species in 2 genera) are restricted to the New World tropics. Only one species occurs as far north as southern Texas and, perhaps, Arizona.

Ghost-Faced Bats

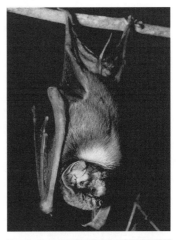

Ghost-faced bats are easily identifiable by the complex folding and ridging of the membranes attached to their lower lips. It's thought that these membranes relax into a funnel-like structure that aids in the capture of insects when the bat is in flight. This may be the source of their name. The neck is so flexible that the head can turn to look straight backward as seen in the photograph. They are locally common in southern Texas, where some examples have been captured in almost every month of the year. In Arizona they have been taken from only one locality in the month of June. A single young, born in late June, is normal.

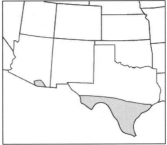

Selected measurements include: total length (nose to tail tip), 3.7 inches (in.) (95 millimeters [mm]); tail, 1 in. (25mm); ear (from notch), 0.6 in. (15mm); forearm, 2 in. (50mm); wingspan, 15 in. (370mm); and weight, 0.5 ounces [oz.] (14 grams [g]).

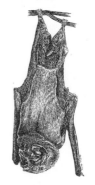

Ghost-Faced Bat,
Family Mormoopidae,
Mormoops megalophylla

NEW WORLD LEAF-NOSED BAT FAMILY
(Phyllostomidae)

*M*embers of this family (143 species in 49 genera) are
restricted to the New World tropics, with 5 species
occurring as far north as the southernmost parts of the Southwest
and in south Florida. Most are medium to large sized and all have
a prominent triangular flap (the "leaf nose") of flesh extending
upward from the tip of the nose.

Leaf-nosed bats are active and require food throughout the
year. Many feed on the nectar, pollen, or fruits of various tropical
and subtropical plants. One group of nectar feeders has an
elongated snout, an extendable tongue, and other features
reminiscent of the adaptations for nectar feeding seen in
hummingbirds. Not surprisingly, they're sometimes called
hummingbird bats. In contrast, fruit-eating species generally have
short snouts, a wide mouth, and strong jaw muscles.

Various other groups of leaf-nosed bats feed on insects they
capture in flight. A few gather a diet of small tree frogs and large
insects from the limbs or leaves of trees.

Because these bats don't hibernate, they must move to new
areas when seasonal food resources become unavailable. Several
undertake significant north-south movements, such as the two
species that are found in the southwestern United States during
the warm months. Others make seasonal migrations up and down
mountain slopes.

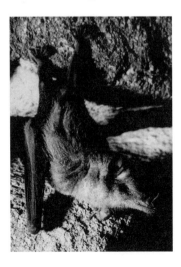
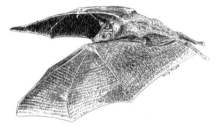

Short-Eared, Nectar-Feeding Bat
Choeronycteris mexicana

Short-Eared, Nectar-feeding Bats

The two major types of leaf-nosed bats are the short-eared, nectar-feeding species, and the big-eared, insect-feeding bats. The first type includes 3 species, arranged in 2 genera. All are essentially tropical New World forms that move into the southern parts of California, Arizona, New Mexico, and the Big Bend region of west Texas during the late spring and summer months.

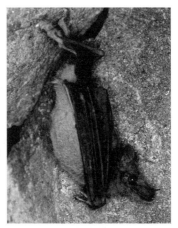

Here they give birth to a single young and feed on the nectar and fruits of various plants, especially organ pipe and saguaro cacti and some agaves (century plants). When this source of food disappears in September and early October, the bats migrate southward to spend the winter and early spring feeding on the flowers and fruits of more tropical plants.

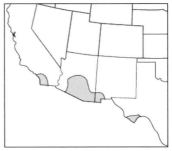

Selected measurements include: total length, 3 to 3.57 in. (75-90mm); tail, 1.6 in. (40mm) or absent; ear, 0.6 in. (16mm); forearm, 2 in. (50mm); wingspan, 13.5 to 16 in. (350-410mm); and weight, 0.4 oz. (18g).

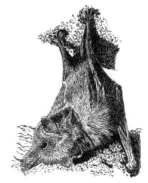

Short-Eared, Nectar-Feeding Bats,
Family Phyllostomidae,
Choeronycteris mexicana and
Choeronycteris leptonycteris

Big-Eared, Insect-feeding Bats

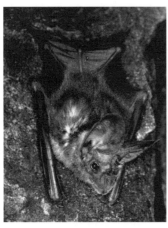

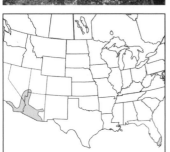

Included in this major type are 2 species of leaf-nosed bats that are members of 2 separate genera. Both feed mainly on insects. One occurs in southern California and Arizona; the other is confined to subtropical south Florida. Neither hibernates but remains in day roosts during unusually cold storms in the winter. The western species feeds mainly on insects; the Florida species feeds on insects as well as fruits, flowers and leaves.

Selected measurements include: total length, 3.5 to 3.8 in. (80-90mm); tail, 1.6 in. (40mm); ear, 0.9 to 1.3 in. (20-33mm); forearm, 2 in. (50mm); wingspan, 13.5 in. (350mm); and weight, 0.4 oz. (12g).

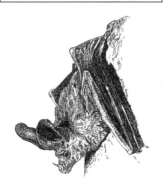

Big-Eared, Insect-Feeding,
Leaf-Nosed Bats,
Family Phyllostomidae,
Macrotus californicus
and *Artibeus jamaicenensis*

PLAIN-NOSED BAT FAMILY
(*Vespertilionidae*)

M embers of this family (80 species in 12 genera) occur almost worldwide from the tree line in the north, to the southern tips of South America, Africa, and Australia.

Most are small to medium in size, feed on a range of insects, and hibernate during the cold parts of the year. Most eat insects they capture in flight. Some can hover and search leaf surfaces to seek and capture insects. A few capture large beetles, grasshoppers, and even scorpions from the surface of the ground.

A few plain-nosed bats have the ability to capture small minnows, shrimp, and other marine life from the surface of gulfs and streams. None of the fish-eating species occur in the United States but one species is found just to the south in the Sea of Cortez (Gulf of California).

In North American north of Mexico there are 29 species grouped in 10 genera. Here we'll look at 6 major groups of plain-nosed bats.

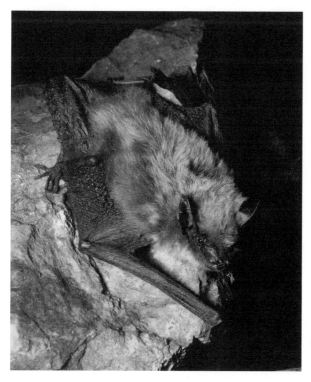

MOUSE-EARED BAT,
Family Vespertilionidae,
genus *Myotis*
(14 species)

Mouse-Eared Bats

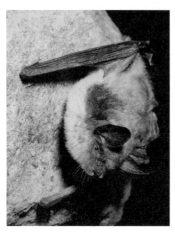

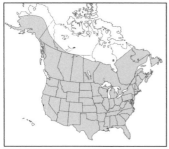

Mouse-eared bats (genus *Myotis*) live in the temperate and tropical climates of both the Old World and the New World. Currently 84 species are recognized in the genus, only 14 of which occur in this area.

This major group includes several small brown bats, including one widely distributed in the United States and Canada called the *little brown bat (Myotis lucifugus)*. All members of the genus have relatively short, mouselike ears, a plain nose, and a tail encased for the full length of the interfemoral membrane (the membrane between the legs).

In the United States any "little brown bat" with these features that also has a relatively long, sharply pointed tragus is a member of this major group. The tragus? Put your finger in your ear. Feel that rounded flap at the front? That's the tragus. In the mouse-eared bats, this is long, thin, and pointed.

Mouse-eared bats vary in size. In the United States, the smallest (California myotis) has a forearm length of about 1.3 in. (32mm), ear length of 0.5 in. (12mm), and a weight of 0.2 oz. (5g). The cave myotis has a forearm length of about 1.6 in. (42mm) and a weight of 0.4 oz. (12g). The long-eared myotis has an ear length of 0.9 in. (22mm).

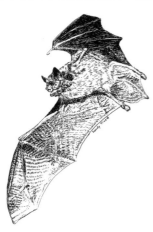

MOUSE-EARED BATS,
Family Vespertilionidae,
genus *Myotis* (14 species)

Big Brown Bats

A single species of the big brown bat occurs in the United States. It is widely distributed across the country, from sea level to the mountains, and from the West Coast to the East Coast. It has been referred to as the *English sparrow* of the bats, because it is so widely distributed and readily takes up residence in human-built structures. It's larger than the mouse-eared bats, thus its common name. The tip of the tragus is broadly rounded.

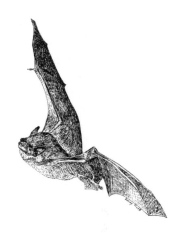

A total of 31 species is known in the genus. These occur in tropical and temperate areas of both the Old World and the New World. In temperate regions, hibernation in the cold months is the way of life.

Selected measurements of the species found in the United States include: total length, 4 in. (102mm); tail, 1.5 in. (39mm); ear, 0.4 in. (11mm); forearm, 1.9 in. (47mm); wingspan, 13.4 in. (340mm); and weight, 0.4 oz. (12g).

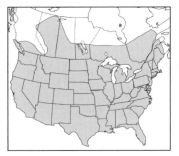

BIG BROWN BAT,
Family Vespertilionidae,
Eptesicus fuscus

Because of their wide distribution, these are among the more commonly seen bats. Not only are they often spotted leaving a roost in some attic and flying around a street light, but they're also found sick on the ground.

Pipistrelles

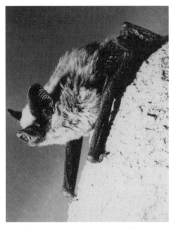

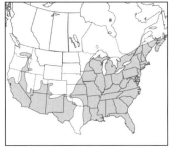

Pipistrelles reside in the tropical and temperate zones of both the Old World and the New World. Fifty different species are currently recognized, only 2 of which occur in North America north of Mexico, one in the West, the other in the East. The western species *(Pipistrellus hesperus)* lives mainly alone or in small groups in rock crevices or on the sides of buildings. It's the smallest of the bats found in the United States; an adult rarely weighs more than a tenth of an ounce.

Pipistrelles fly early in the evening, shortly after sundown. Thus, they're probably the most commonly seen bat in their range. They flit about, feeding on small insects.

Selected measurements include: total length, 2.8 to 3.2 in. (72-80mm); tail, 1.3 to 1.5 in. (32-36mm); ear, 0.5 in. (12mm); forearm, 1.2 to 1.3 in. (32-34mm); wingspan, 8 to 9 in. (210-230mm); and weight, 0.1 to 0.3 oz. (3-6g).

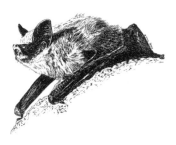

PIPISTRELLES,
Family Vespertilionidae,
genus *Pipistrellus* (2 species)

Evening Bats

The pipistrelle found in the eastern United States, from the Great Lakes southward to the Gulf of Mexico, is the evening bat. Seven species of this bat are known, living in geographically separate areas. One group is found in Australia and adjacent New Guinea; another lives in southwestern Arabia and much of East Africa. A few are also found in Cuba and the northeastern coastal areas of Mexico just south of Texas.

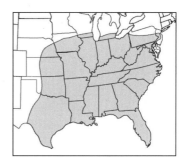

EVENING BAT,
Family Vespertilionidae,
Nycticeius humeralis

To most of us the U.S. evening bat looks like just another mouse-eared bat with a short, rounded tragus. The difference is that it has only two upper incisors between the canine teeth in contrast to the four that occur in other bats. However, most of us are not thrilled with the thought of asking a bat to say "aah" so we can count its teeth, so identification is difficult.

Selected measurements include: total length, 3.5 in. (90mm); tail, 1.6 in. (42mm); ear, 0.5 in. (12mm); forearm, 1.5 in. (38mm); wingspan, 10.6 in. (270mm); and weight, 0.4 oz. (12g).

TREE BATS

Four of the major types in the plain-nosed bat family can be usefully grouped as the "tree bat" type. Most of the other members of the family are "cave bats."

Cave bats spend the daylight hours in a dark roost. Such roosts vary with kind of bat, season of the year, and even with different genders and individuals. They can be found in a dark hollow in a tree, a deep crevice in a rock, the attic or another cavity in a building, in an actual cave, or in a mine tunnel—in other words, in almost any dark, cavelike place that is relatively hard for a predator to reach. Most cave bats gather in small to large groups.

In contrast, the tree bats rarely enter such a roost. Instead, they hang, often singly, in a clump of leaves on a tree or in some indentation in the bark of a tree. Compared to their cave bat relatives, tree bats have denser, longer fur, especially noticeable on the interfemoral membranes.

All tree bats feed on flying insects, which are only available during warm weather. Most make an annual migration, spending summers as far north as Canada, and winters in the southern United States or in Mexico.

Because they roost in trees and migrate seasonally through unfamiliar areas, tree bats are more commonly encountered on the ground than are cave bats. As a result, the number that ends up in the health laboratory for rabies testing is high.

While cave bats rarely have more than a single offspring each year, tree bats generally have two (even three or four) young in the annual litter. This tells you something about the difference in their rates of survival as species. The following four major groups are all tree bats.

Silver-Haired Bats

Among the bats of this region, these are uniquely colored. Their fur is black but the tips of many of the hairs are white. The result is a silvery appearance. Like other tree bats, the silver-haired bat has dense and relatively long fur, especially on the interfemoral membrane.

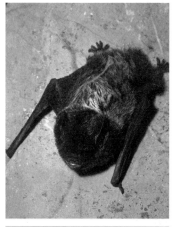

During the summer, most female silver-haired bats migrate from the southern parts of the United States northward into states from Maine to Washington and the tree-covered portions of Canada. There the young (one or two per litter) are born in late June or early July. Males also move northward, but usually not as far north as the females.

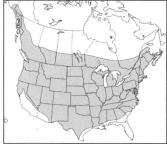

Selected measurements include: total length, 4 in. (102mm); tail, 1.7 in. (43mm); ear, 0.6 in. (16mm); forearm, 1.6 in. (42mm); wingspan, 11.8 in. (300mm); and weight, 0.4 oz. (10g).

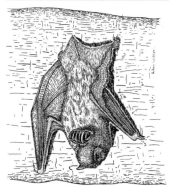

SILVER-HAIRED BAT,
Family Vespertilionidae,
Lasionycteris noctivagans

Hoary Bats

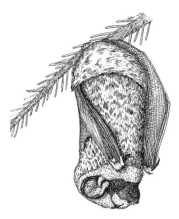

This large bat is a strong flyer. It is capable of making an annual north-south migration from southern Canada to the southern United States and even on southward into central Mexico.

The back is yellowish to dark brown in color with many of the hairs tipped in white. The result is a hoary or aged appearance. Its gray fur blends in well with clumps of leaves and the branches of trees where it spends the day.

Selected measurements include: total length, 5.6 in. (142mm); tail, 1.9 in. (49mm); ear, 0.7 in. (17mm); forearm, 2.1 in. (53mm); wingspan, 15.8 in. (400mm); and weight, 1 oz. (28g).

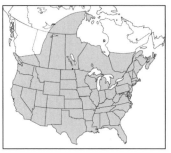

HOARY BAT,
Family Vespertilionidae,
Lasiurus cinereus

Red Bats

Red bats vary in color from bright orange-red to buff-yellow, with some hairs tipped in white. The hairs on the arms, legs, and interfemoral membrane are thick and long. Most of the members of this group found in the eastern United States and Canada are a brighter red than those in the Southwest. Like other tree bats, they migrate seasonally, spending winters in the south and summers in the north. In the western states (New Mexico, Arizona, and southern California) most migrate on southward into Mexico for the winter. In northern California they migrate from the mountains down into the foothills and central valleys.

The females give birth to two to four young in late June or early July. The mother and young hang, blending in with vegetation as a cluster of leaves, or even looking like a ripe peach hanging in a peach tree.

Selected measurements include: total length, 4.3 in. (108mm); tail, 1.7 in. (43mm); ear, 0.4 in. (10mm); forearm, 1.7 in. (42mm); wingspan, 11.8 in. (300mm); and weight, 0.4 oz. (12g).

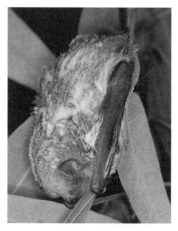

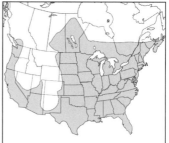

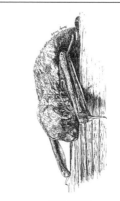

RED BATS,
Family Vespertilionidae, *Lasiurus borealis* and *Lasiurus seminolus*

Yellow Bats

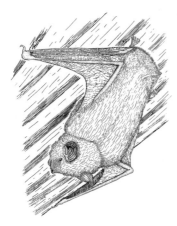

The yellow bats are slightly larger than the red bats. They differ in color, being yellowish to buff and with only a few white-tipped hairs. Like other tree bats, they have unusually long, thick hair on the interfemoral membrane and limbs.

Yellow bats are essentially restricted to the southernmost parts of the United States and southward into Central America. A common roost site is among the dead fronds of palm trees.

Selected measurements include: total length, 4.4 in. (110mm); tail, 2 in. (50mm); ear, 0.6 in. (16mm); forearm, 2 in. (50mm); wingspan, 14.8 in. (370mm); and weight, 0.5 oz. (13g).

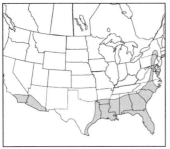

YELLOW BATS,
Family Vespertilionidae,
Lasiurus intermedius
and *Lasiurus ega*

Big-Eared Bats

Big-eared bats, also known as *lump-nosed bats,* are relatively small. They have exceptionally long ears that curl around in a ram's horn shape as the bat sleeps. The tragus (see page 68) is unusually long. The wings are wide and the almost naked interfemoral membrane is long.

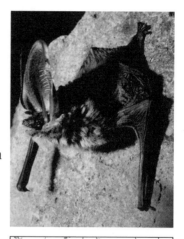

These bats are agile fliers. They can hover over the leaf of a plant and search its surface for insect food with echo-locating sonarlike beeps. Their roosts are usually in caves or mine tunnels, but in summer they sometimes roost in attics.

Selected measurements include: total length, 3.9 in. (100mm); tail, 1.8 in. (45mm); ear, 1.4in. (35 mm); forearm, 1.2 in. (30mm); wingspan, 11.8 in. (300mm); and weight, 0.4 oz. (9g).

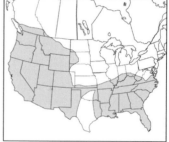

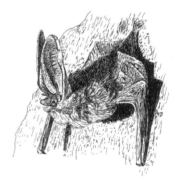

BIG-EARED BATS,
Family Vespertilionidae,
Plecotus townsendii
and *Plecotus rafinesquii*

Spotted Bats

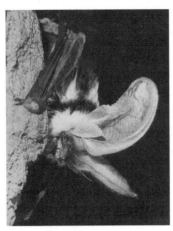

This rare plain-nosed bat has unique, extremely large, pink-colored ears and black fur with three obvious white spots on the back, one on each shoulder and one on the rump.

Selected measurements include: total length, 4.4 in. (110mm); tail, 1.9 in. (48mm); ear, 1.8 in. (44mm); forearm, 2 in. (50mm); wingspan, 13.5 in. (345mm); and weight, 1.8 oz. (44g).

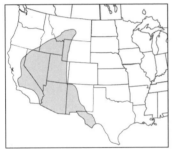

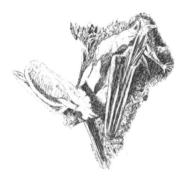

SPOTTED BAT,
Family Vespertilionidae,
Euderma maculatum

Allen's Big-Eared Bats

This is another big-eared bat known only from scattered localities in the western United States. It appears to be an inhabitant of rocky cliffs.

Selected measurements include: total length, 4.4 in. (112mm); tail, 2 in. (50mm); ear, 1.5 in. (40mm); forearm, 1.9 in. (48mm); wingspan, 13.4 in. (340mm); and weight, 0.45 oz. (13g).

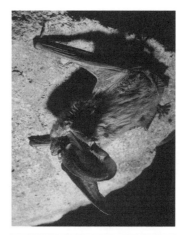

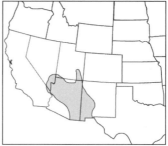

ALLEN'S BIG-EARED BAT,
Family Vespertilionidae,
Idionycteris phyllotis

Pallid Bats

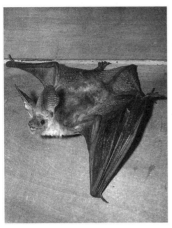

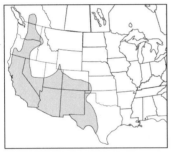

The pallid type of big-eared bat is relatively large and quite sturdy. It feeds on a variety of large insects, such as beetles, moths, grasshoppers, and even scorpions, which they take from the surface of the ground. The bat takes its prey to a night roost, which is often in a shallow rock overhang, or even on a porch or in a carport. There it eats the soft parts of the insect and drops the wings, legs, and other hard parts.

During the summer, pallid bats roost by day in attics, railroad or highway bridges, and similar places. Little is known of their winter habitats. Most probably spend the winter in small groups in small rock crevices. One or two young are born in June.

Selected measurements include: total length, 4.7 in. (120mm); tail, 1.8 in. (46mm); ear, 1.2 in. (30mm); forearm, 2.2 in. (58mm); wingspan, 14.9 in. (380mm); and weight, 0.7 oz. (20g).

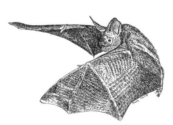

PALLID BAT,
Family Vespertilionidae,
Antrozous pallidus

Free-Tailed Bat Family
(*Molossidae*)

*M*embers of this mainly tropical family of bats occur in both the Old World and the New World. About 80 species, grouped in 12 genera, are currently recognized. All are insect feeders. Most are adapted for day roosting in cracks and crevices of rocks and buildings. One of their favorite roosting sites is under roofing tiles.

The 6 species (from 3 genera) found in the United States occur mostly in the southern states. There are 3 major types, each corresponding to one of the 3 genera.

Brazilian Free-Tailed Bats

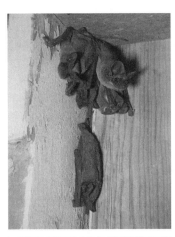

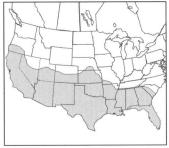

This bat is also known as the *Mexican free-tailed bat* and as the *guano bat*. They earned the latter common name because of the huge accumulations of bat guano found in the extremely large maternity colonies that reside in caves during the summer.

During the migration seasons (May to June and August to September), they make their transient roosts in buildings, crevices in bridges, and similar places where they often come into contact with humans and pets.

Selected measurements include: total length, 4.0 in. (100mm); tail, 1.3 in. (34mm); ear, 0.7 in. (17mm); forearm, 1.7 in. (40mm); wingspan, 11.9 in. (300mm); and weight, 0.4 oz. (12g).

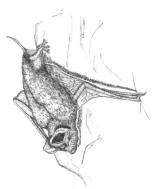

BRAZILIAN FREE-TAILED BAT,
Family Molossidae,
Tadarida braziliensis

Large Free-Tailed Bats

In the United States these larger relatives of the Brazilian free-tailed bat are restricted to the southwestern states. Most occur to the south, in Mexico. In the southernmost parts of the United States they appear to live throughout the year, leaving the winter hibernation during warm periods to forage on any available insects.

Selected measurements include: total length, 4.1 to 5.1 in. (110-130mm); tail, 1.6 to 2 in. (42-50mm); ear, 0.8 to 1.1 in. (20-27mm); forearm, 1.4 to 1.9 in. (48-60mm); wingspan, 13.8 to 17 in. (350-430mm); and weight, 0.5 to 0.9 oz. (16-25g).

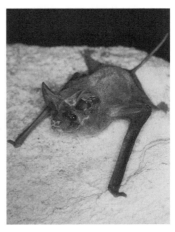

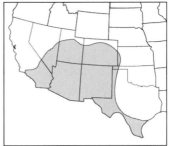

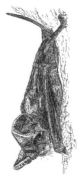

LARGE FREE-TAILED BATS,
Family Molossidae,
Nyctinomops femorosaccus
and *Nyctinomops macrotis*

Mastiff Bats

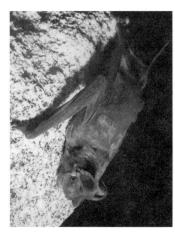

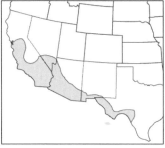

This type of free-tailed bat is the largest of the bat residents of the United States. One species *(Eumops perotis)* has a wingspread of almost 21 in. Day roosts are in small colonies with up to 50 or 60 individuals, located in rock crevices high on a cliff face or in similar places in tall buildings.

The wings are long and narrow; the flight is swift and strong. Food consists of large flying insects. The mastiff bats take water from large pools and streams where a long stretch of smooth-surfaced water is available.

Selected measurements of the larger, more widely distributed species include: total length, 7.2 in. (185mm); tail, 2.4 in. (60mm); ear, 1.6 in. (41mm); forearm, 3.1 in. (80mm); wingspan, 22 in. (560mm); and weight, 2.1 oz. (60g). The other two species are almost as large, with forearms ranging from 2.6 to 3 in. (65-75mm).

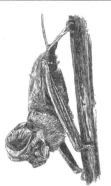

MASTIFF BATS,
Family Molossidae,
genus *Eumops* (3 species)

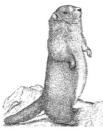

RODENTS (Order Rodentia)

Rodents are much more diverse than the bats or the hares and rabbits. Currently, 4,629 living species of mammals are recognized in the world. These are usually grouped in 1,135 genera, 135 families, in 26 orders. Of these, 2,015 species are rodents (443 genera, 28 families).

In the United States and Canada about 199 species of rodents are known (39 genera, 8 families). For our purposes here, these 199 species are arranged in 28 different "major types" that can usually be recognized as having obvious distinctions. For example, most novices have little difficulty seeing the differences between a kangaroo rat and a pack rat, or a chipmunk and a tree squirrel, even though they may have never seen or heard of these mammals. Such species are easy to recognize.

In contrast, even professional mammalogists often have difficulty quickly distinguishing among a cliff chipmunk, a California chipmunk, a long-eared chipmunk, and other kinds of chipmunks. Because all chipmunks are very similar in size, shape and color, only close attention to minor differences reveals that they are different species.

The eight families of rodents in the United States and Canada are:

Mountain Beaver Family
(Aplodontidae—1 species, 1 major type)

Squirrel Family
(Sciuridae—62 species, 8 major types)

North American Burrowing Rodent Family
(Geomyidae—13 species, 1 major type)

Beaver Family
(Castoridae—1 species, 1 major type)

North American Desert Rodent Family
(Heteromyidae—36 species, 4 major types)

Rats and Mice Family
(Muridae—51 species, 10 major types)

Jumping Mice and Rats Family
(Dipodidae—4 species, 1 major type)

Porcupine Family
(Erethizontidae—1 species, 1 major type)

To help you distinguish among the species grouped here as major groups, several useful references are given.

MOUNTAIN BEAVER FAMILY
(Aplodontidae)

The mountain beaver, sometimes known by the Native American name of Sewellel, is the only living species in this family. Even as fossils they are only known in western North America. At present they're restricted to moist habitats in northern California, Oregon, Washington and British Columbia where they live in underground burrows.

Mountain Beavers

Mountain beavers are modified for living in an underground tunnel. The body is chunky; the limbs, tail and ears are short; the eyes are small. The limbs are stout and the short toes have strong claws. All of these adaptations make for an efficient digging machine.

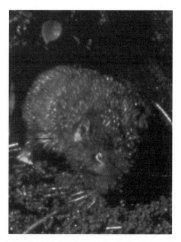

The short, dense fur is about the same color on the back as on the belly, ranging from cinnamon to brown with older individuals becoming grayish.

Their common name probably resulted because their fur resembles that of the beaver. They certainly don't live in streams and have none of the adaptive features of the beaver.

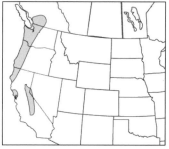

Body size is about that of an adult muskrat. Average adult measurements are: total length (nose to tail tip), 18 in. (450mm); tail, 1.5 in. (40mm); hind foot, 2 in. (50mm); ear, 1 in. (25mm); and weight, 2.2 lb. (1 kilogram [kg]). Females are about 10 percent smaller than males.

Mountain beaver burrows are up to 10 in. (250mm) in diameter and may be up to 300 feet in length. These rodents are active throughout the year, especially at night, and rarely leave their burrows. They feed on the roots, stems and leaves of a wide variety of plants. In March or April a litter of two or three blind young is born in a grass-lined nest.

To date, there have been no reports of this animal serving as a reservoir for human diseases.

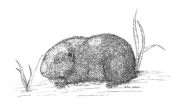

MOUNTAIN BEAVER,
Family Aplodontidae,
species *Aplodontia rufa*

SQUIRREL FAMILY
(Sciuridae)

The squirrel family includes about 251 different living species (15 percent of all living rodents) that are grouped into 49 genera. These are divided into two subfamilies: flying squirrels (Petauristinae) and the tree and ground squirrels (Sciurinae). Flying squirrels are active only at night and apparently never hibernate. Members of the subfamily Sciurinae are divided into a number of tribes. All ground and tree squirrels are active during the day, and several kinds hibernate for long periods of the year.

The 62 different species of squirrel present in the United States and Canada can be easily grouped into 8 major types: flying squirrel (2 species), marmot (4 species), prairie dogs (4 species), ground squirrels (17 species), antelope squirrels (4 species), chipmunks (22 species), chipmunk squirrels (2 species), and tree squirrels (7 species).

SUBFAMILY PTEROMYINAE

This subfamily occurs in Europe, Asia and North America. Fourteen genera are recognized, only one of which occurs in North America. The largest is the Giant flying squirrel of Asia— total length, 4ft. (1.2 m); weight 4.5 pounds (2kg). The North American species are among the smallest in the subfamily

Flying Squirrels

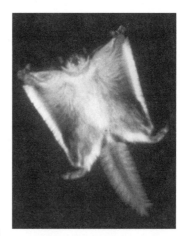

The fur-covered gliding membrane between the fore and hind legs and soft, silky fur are unique to flying squirrels. Their tail is bushy, broad, and flattened; their ears small. The back is brownish in color; the tail, blackish above; the belly, white to creamy white.

A typical adult measures: total length, 12.6 in. (320mm); tail, 5.5 in. (140mm); hind foot, 1.7 in. (42mm); ear, 1.1 in. (28mm); and weight, 5.6 oz. (160g).

Flying squirrels are most common in dense coniferous forests where they're active at night throughout the year. Food includes seeds, nuts, fungi, berries, insects, and even small birds. Nests are constructed of shredded bark in hollow trees. Sometimes they build a roof over an abandoned bird nest and use it as a retreat. After a gestation period of 40 days, the female bears a litter of two to five young in May or June.

Spotted fever and rabies have been reported in flying squirrels. It has been suggested that the flying squirrel may have been infected with rabies by the bite of a rabid bat.

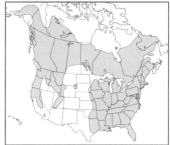

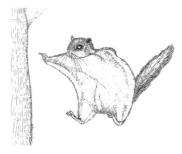

FLYING SQUIRREL,
Family Sciuridae,
Subfamily Pteromyinae
genus *Glaucomys* (2 species)

Subfamily Sciurinae

This subfamily contains eight subgroups, known as *tribes,* three of which occur in the U.S. and Canada: Marmotini (Holarctic ground squirrels), Tamiasciurini (chipmunk squirrels), and Sciurini (tree squirrels). All are active during the day.

Holarctic Ground Squirrels
(Tribe Marmotini)

Members of this tribe are widely distributed in Europe, Asia, and North America. They're called *Holarctic* after the northern regions in which they live.

Most Holarctic ground squirrels feed mainly or entirely on moist new plant growth (buds, berries, fruits, stems, leaves, roots). Some, especially chipmunks, also include nuts, insects, bird eggs, and small animals in their diets. It is a diverse group, with about 73 species, arranged in 5 genera, usually being recognized. In the United States and Canada there are 39 species, grouped in 5 genera.

Like other members of the subfamily, Holarctic ground squirrels are active during the day. A *holarctic* distribution is totally around the arctic region of both the old and new world. Most hibernate during part of the year. Major types that occur in this area include marmots, prairie dogs, ground squirrels, antelope ground squirrels and chipmunks.

Marmots (Groundhogs)

Marmots occur in Europe, northern Asia, and northern North America. About 14 species are known, four of which live in the United States. Marmots are large, heavy-set, ground squirrel-shaped animals with small ears and a short tail. Their general body shape has been adapted for burrowing in the ground. Color is usually tan or brownish, often washed with white, and includes an obvious white patch between the eyes.

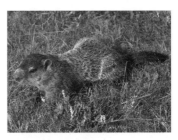

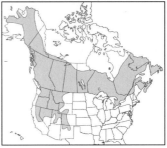

Typical measurements of the North American species include: total length, 23.6 in. (600mm); tail, 8 in. (200mm); hind foot, 3.2 in. (80mm); ear, 1 in. (25mm); and weight, to 20 lb. (9kg). Individuals vary from these measurements by up to 15 percent, in part because growth continues after they reach adult status.

Marmots—also called *groundhogs* and *woodchucks*—are usually found in rocky places in the mountains, often along road cuts. There they feed on various plants, especially grasses, that are readily available only during the short summer. Marmots store a great amount of body fat which maintains them during the long, winter hibernation. Usually they lose about half their body weight during hibernation.

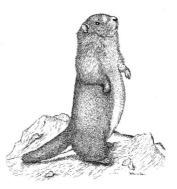

MARMOTS (Groundhogs), Family Sciuridae, Subfamily Sciurinae, Tribe Marmotini, genus *Marmota* (4 species)

They reach adult size in the third year, even though some females have young in their second year. A dominant male defends a territory of about 1.5 acres (0.6 hectares) from other males. Several females and young may live in this territory. A litter of four or five young is common.

Diseases isolated from marmots include Colorado tick fever, rabies, Lyme disease, Rocky Mountain spotted fever, leptospirosis, murine typhus, plague and tularemia.

Prairie Dogs

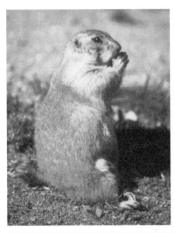

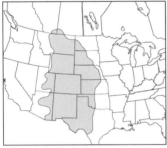

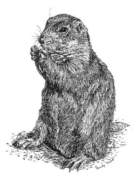

PRAIRIE DOGS,
Family Sciuridae,
Subfamily Sciurinae,
Tribe Marmotini,
genus *Cynomys* (4 species)

Prairie dogs are found only in open grasslands of western North America. There are 5 species, 4 of which occur in the United States. All are grouped in a single genus. Their body weight is about that of a large tree squirrel, but the shape is chunky and the tail and ears are short. The short, white-tipped tail has a mid-dorsal gray streak (along the back). The prairie dog's fur is light in color, usually uniformly buff, above and below.

Typical measurements of an adult are: total length, 13.8 in. (350mm); tail, 2.4 in. (60mm); hind foot, 2.2 in. (55mm); ear, 0.5 in. (12mm); and weight, 2 lb. (900g).

Prairie dogs live in colonies of 200 or more. Some colonies number in the thousands and cover several square miles. They have a complex social system with various divisions, termed *wards*.

Prairie dogs have an interesting communication system. They "talk" to each other by calls, body position (such as tail up, tail down), and odors. They use these means to tell each other about such events as a hawk flying nearby (danger to all), or to tell stranger prairie dogs to leave the neighborhood.

Their food consists of various plant materials, especially short grasses. Roots, bulbs, worms, and insects are also eaten. Winter months are spent in hibernation.

Plague is the only disease that has been isolated in prairie dogs.

Ground Squirrels

Ground squirrels occur in Europe, northern Asia, and North America. They're a diverse group. About 36 different species are known, with 17 species occurring in the United States and Canada, mostly in the western states and provinces. In one local region, it's not unusual to find 3 or more species, each living in a different habitat (such as sandy soil, clay soil, or a rocky area).

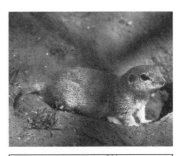

All ground squirrels are active during the day and, even in warm areas, all hibernate during the winter months. Their activity usually takes place on the ground but most ground squirrels can climb low bushes and cacti.

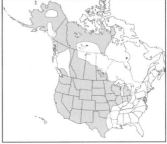

In this area they range in length from about 9 in. (23cm) (about chipmunk size) to 19 in. (48cm) (the size of a tree squirrel). All have the general squirrel appearance, but with short, rounded ears. Some look like chipmunks, with dark and light stripes on the back and a bushy tail, but they don't have stripes on their faces. Ground squirrels' tails vary in length, depending on the size of the body, and from short-haired to bushy. Their dorsal (back) color varies from uniform to spotted, striped, or grizzled. The field guides listed in the references section can help you determine the species you're concerned with.

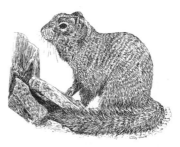

GROUND SQUIRRELS,
Family Sciuridae,
Subfamily Sciurinae,
Tribe Marmotini,
genus *Spermophilus* (17 species)

Typical measurements for a small ground squirrel are: total length, 9.3 in. (235mm); tail, 3 in. (75mm); hind foot, 1.3 in. (33mm); ear, 0.4 in.

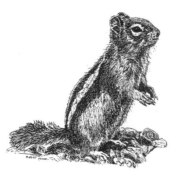

(10mm); and weight, 4.6 oz. (130g). The larger species typically measure: total length, 19 in. (475mm); tail, 8 in. (200mm); hind foot, 2.4 in. (60mm); ear, 1.2 in. (30mm); and weight, 1.7 lb. (760g).

Most species of ground squirrels are found in grassy areas where they live in underground burrows that rarely show any sign of a mound at the entrances. Food consists of seeds, green plants, and many insects. Hibernation may last five to six months. They mate in the spring, and a litter of 5 to 13 young is born in an underground nest.

Diseases isolated from ground squirrels include Colorado tick fever, encephalitis, Rocky Mountain spotted fever, murine typhus, plague and tularemia.

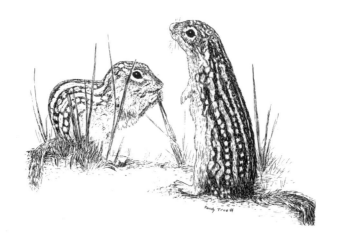

Antelope Squirrels

In North America, antelope squirrels are known only in the southwestern United States and adjacent Mexico. Four species occur here, each slightly larger than a chipmunk.

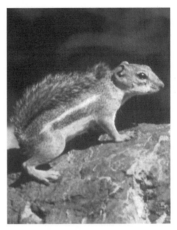

Antelope squirrels are easy to distinguish from other small squirrel-like rodents by a well-developed white stripe that extends on each side from the shoulder to the hip. They have no central dark stripe. The bushy tail is usually held curved over the back, exposing the white undersurface. Unlike chipmunks, they have no stripes on the sides of the face. They are probably called *antelope squirrels* because their fur color is almost the same as that of the pronghorn antelope.

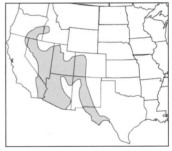

Typical measurements are: total length, 9.1 in. (230mm); tail, 3 in. (75mm); hind foot, 1.5 in. (38mm); ear, 0.5 in. (12mm); and weight, 4.4 oz. (125g).

Antelope squirrels are restricted to desert and desert grassland habitats. They're active in daytime during most of the year. On cold winter days they remain underground. On hot summer days they are most active in the early morning. Food consists of seeds, berries, fruits, insects, and green vegetation. Buds and new growth of mesquite and various cactus fruits are seasonal favorites. They use several short, shallow burrows for protection from heat and enemies as well as for food storage. In the early spring a litter (five to nine young) is born in an underground nest chamber.

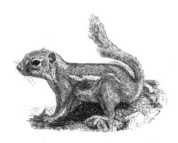

ANTELOPE SQUIRRELS,
Family Sciuridae, Subfamily Sciurinae,
Tribe Marmotini,
genus *Ammospermophilus*
(4 species)

Surprisingly, no human diseases have been noted as being found in antelope squirrels. Probably they have about the same diseases as the ground squirrels.

Chipmunks

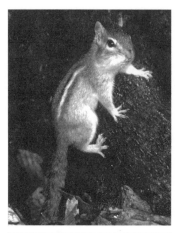

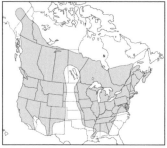

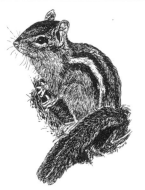

CHIPMUNKS,
Family Sciuridae, Subfamily Sciurinae,
Tribe Marmotini,
genus *Tamias* (22 species)

The chipmunk is a type of ground squirrel that occurs in Europe, northern Asia, and North America, with at least 25 different species currently recognized. Of these, about 22 occur in the United States and Canada. Several of these "species" have very limited distribution. The western species, until recently, was placed in the genus *Eutamias.* Now all *Eutamias* are considered to be a subgenus in the genus *Tamias.*

Chipmunks are active during the day. Most live on the ground, generally on the edges of forests.

What distinguishes a chipmunk is its stripes. A chipmunk has five long black stripes on the back and three short black stripes on each side of the head. The tail is long and bushy. The belly is usually buff, bright orange, or grayish yellow. The ears are relatively long and pointed.

Typical measurements are: total length, 7.7 in. (195mm); tail, 3.5 in. (90mm); hind foot, 1.2 in. (30mm); ear, 0.6 in. (16mm); and weight, 1.8 oz. (50g).

The chipmunk's food consists of many kinds of seeds, berries, fungi, and other plant material. In some areas they also eat juniper berries, acorns, pine nuts, and some insects. Four to six young per litter are common, and some females have two litters in a year. They store various seeds in underground burrows, and spend most of the cold season in hibernation.

Chipmunks have been reported as reservoirs for hanta virus pulmonary syndrome, Rocky Mountain spotted fever, encephalitis, Lyme disease, plague and relapsing fever.

CHIPMUNK SQUIRRELS
(Tribe Tamiasciurini)

The chipmunk squirrels have features of their anatomy that are intermediate between those of tree squirrels and chipmunks, thus their common name. Chipmunk squirrels are a small group with discontinuous distribution: some in China and others in North America.

The 4 known living species are grouped into 2 genera, the chickarees or red squirrels of North America, and the Chinese rock squirrels of parts of mainland China. They're about half the size of a tree squirrel, weighing between 140 and 300 grams.

Chipmunk squirrels spend much of their time on the ground and behave very much the same as chipmunks, except for climbing. The North American red squirrels readily climb trees, while the Chinese rock squirrels climb on rocky exposures in forested areas. None of the chipmunk squirrels hibernates.

Red Squirrels

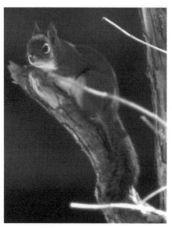

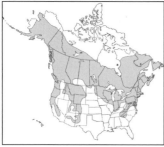

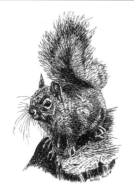

RED SQUIRRELS,
Family Sciuridae, Subfamily Sciurinae,
Tribe Tamiasciurini, genus
Tamiasciurus (2 species)

Two species of red squirrels live in the United States. Both have a short black stripe along the lateral edge of the whitish to yellowish belly. The tail is narrow and shorter than the head and body. Black-tipped hairs occur along the edge and on the tip of the tail. Red squirrels are usually heard before they are seen. Their "bark" or "chatter" is given, perhaps as a warning cry to others, as soon as they see you or some other potential danger.

Typical measurements are: total length, 12.8 in. (325mm); tail, 4.9 in. (125mm); hind foot, 1.9 in. (50mm); ear, 1 in. (25mm); and weight, 8.1 oz. (250g).

Red squirrels live in coniferous forests, especially among spruces and firs at higher elevations. Even though they're active in the day throughout the year, they usually remain in their nests during cold stormy weather. In summers most activity takes place in the morning.

Their food includes fungi, nuts, and seeds. They often carry food to a "feeding stump" where they watch the surroundings as they extract the edible parts from nuts or cones. After some time, a huge stack of debris accumulates there.

Red squirrels make their nests in hollow trees or build them of twigs and bark high in the tree. Two litters of two to seven young each are born, one in April or May and another as late as September.

Red squirrels haven't been reported as serving as reservoirs for any of human diseases. Some diseases have probably been found in individuals that were misidentified as "tree squirrels."

TREE SQUIRRELS
(Tribe Sciurini)

The third tribe of nonflying squirrels consists of the tree squirrels, which are restricted to Eurasia and the Americas. African and Oriental tree squirrels belong to different tribes. The Sciurini tribe includes 37 species that are grouped into 5 genera.

Most of these squirrels readily climb trees and some are rarely seen on the ground. All are active during the day on all but the coldest, stormiest days of the year. Their bushy tail is about the same length as the head and body.

Tree Squirrels

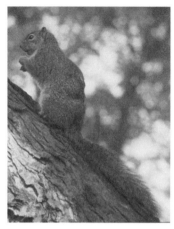

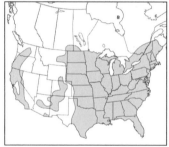

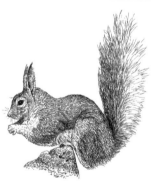

TREE SQUIRRELS,
Family Sciuridae, Subfamily Sciurinae,
Tribe Sciurini, genus *Sciurus*
(7 species)

Five species of tree squirrels, all in the same genus, occur in the United States and Canada. They vary in color; some have tassels on the ears and some don't. In all species, the tail is long and bushy.

Typical measurements are: total length, 22 in. (550mm); tail, 10.5 in. (270mm); hind foot, 3.2 in. (80mm); ear, 1.2 in. (30mm); and weight, 1 lb. (453g).

Obviously, tree squirrels are restricted to woodland areas. Each species has a preferred type of forest. The eastern fox squirrels and Nayarit fox squirrels mainly inhabit deciduous forests. Arizona gray squirrels live in oak woodlands; Abert's squirrels in areas of Ponderosa pine; and the Western gray squirrel in coastal oak woodlands. In mountainous interior regions they occur in both oak woodlands and redwood forests.

Tree squirrels are active throughout the year, especially in the early morning and late afternoon. During cold, stormy periods they remain in their nests for days at a time. Their food consists of a range of plant materials including leaf buds, flowers, herbs, fungi, berries, pine cones, and acorns. They construct bulky nests of shredded bark and twigs high in trees, or use nests in hollow trees. A litter of one to three young is born in the spring.

Diseases isolated from tree squirrels include encephalitis, Rocky Mountain spotted fever, leptospirosis, murine typhus, plague, relapsing fever and tularemia.

NORTH AMERICAN BURROWING RODENTS
(*Geomyidae*)

*B*iologists have made the interesting discovery that various unrelated rodents have independently evolved in different parts of the world to build and live in underground tunnels, also called *burrows*. In North America, these fossorial rodents evolved from squirrel-like ancestors into the group known as *pocket gophers*. About 34 living species are known, generally grouped in 5 genera. Of these, 8 species, in 3 genera, are generally recognized in this area.

Pocket Gophers

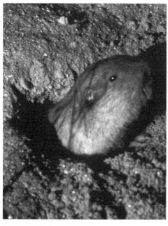

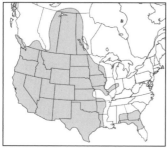

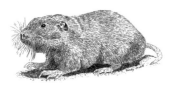

POCKET GOPHERS
3 genera (13 species)

A pocket gopher is about the size of a large, chunky chipmunk. The head is wide, flattened, and wedge-shaped, and the neck is short. The limbs are short, and the forefeet have elongated claws adapted for digging. The ears are tiny, and the tail short and almost hairless.

Pocket gophers get their name from their fur-lined cheek pouches. These pockets, external to the mouth proper, are used to transport food. Those that live in dry areas have light-colored fur, while those in moist regions are almost black.

Measurements of a typical adult are: total length, 9.5 in. (240mm); tail, 3 in. (75mm); hind foot, 1.3 in. (32mm); ear, 0.4 in. (10mm); and weight, 6.7 oz. (190g). They may vary from these specifications by as much as 25 percent. Pocket gophers that live in deep soils are usually larger, while species in areas of rocky soils are usually small.

Pocket gophers are found mainly in soft soils from sea level to high mountain meadows. Alfalfa fields are favored sites. All feed mainly on the roots and bulbs of plants they encounter in their underground feeding tunnels, but at times they pull whole plants down into the burrow and eat leaves, stems and all. They are active throughout the year and may be active at any time of the day or night.

Pocket gophers build a nest in a deep tunnel, often under a rock or the roots of a bush or tree. Generally only one gopher occupies a tunnel system and one system may have 20 or more earth mounds on the surface. They have litters of two to ten, and one or two litters each year are normal.

Like the underground-dwelling mountain beaver, no pocket gophers have been implicated as serving as reservoirs of any human diseases.

BEAVER FAMILY
(*Castoridae*)

This family includes only 2 living species, both grouped in a single genus. One species is restricted to the Old World, the other to North America. Beavers were once widely distributed throughout Europe, northern Asia, and northern North America. As a result of extensive fur trapping, they were eliminated in England and most of the rest of the range by the nineteenth century. Much of the North American range is being restocked.

These large rodents, second in size only to the South American capybara, are noted for their adaptations for life in and around water and their constructions of dams and complex "lodges."

Beavers

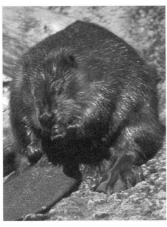

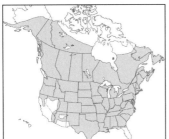

The beaver's adaptations for living in and near water include: webbed hind feet, small ears and a large, flattened, scale-covered tail. All of these help them swim. The pelage, or coat, is long, dense, and water-repellent. The eyes are small and have a nictitating membrane protecting the eye when they are under water. Both the nostrils and the external ear openings can be closed to the water.

Typical measurements are: total length, 38 in. (980mm); tail, 16 in. (406mm); hind foot, 6.7 in. (170mm); ear, 1.3 in. (32mm); and weight, 50 lb. (23kg).

Beavers live in or along permanent streams and lakes that are bordered by trees. They generally live in family groups. Their food consists of the bark and outer layers of various bushes and trees, especially aspens, birches and willows. They have litters of two to eight kits in April or May.

Diseases isolated from beavers include leptospirosis, tularemia and giardiasis.

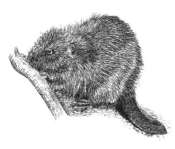

BEAVER,
Family Castoridae,
genus *Castor canadensis,*
American beaver

NORTH AMERICAN DESERT RODENT FAMILY
(*Heteromyidae*)

In the evolutionary history of rodents, the desert family has developed rather recently. Geographically, most deserts aren't interconnected; thus each represents an "island" of new habitat. As a result, no one group of rodents has developed special features for living in the desert climates of Africa, Asia, Australia, South America and North America. Rather, such modifications came about independently in the different deserts in relatively unrelated groups. As a result, rodents of various families are adapted for desert life.

In North America the desert rats belong to the family Heteromyidae. This family includes about 62 living species that are grouped in 6 genera. Like the members of the family Geomyidae (burrowing rodents) they have external, fur-lined cheek pouches. Most have elongated hind feet and legs and a long tail that they use in a jumping type of locomotion. This is an efficient way to move in the open areas of desert and desert grasslands.

American desert rats are small to medium in size, ranging from 50 to 180mm in head and body length, from 45 to 210mm in length of tail, and from 8 to 140 grams in weight.

The heteromyid rodents are, primitively, animals of the warm subtropical and tropical forests that have successfully invaded the semiarid grasslands and the arid Great American Desert. Living members are divided into three subfamilies, two of which have representatives in this area: Perognathinae, with 3 genera and Dipodominae, with 1 genus.

Subfamily Perognathinae — Pocket Mice

The different types of pocket mice are modified in a variety of ways for saltatorial (hopping) locomotion. The auditory bullae—large, hollow outgrowths of the tympanic bone, the bone that surrounds and holds the tympanic membrane (ear drum)—vary from well inflated to extremely inflated. In the Kangaroo mice and most of the Kangaroo rats these are so inflated that up to half of the skull is made up of the two auditory (or tympanic) bullae. As a result, the posterior part of the skull is very wide and flat, giving a wedge-shaped appearance to the skull (see below). Habitats range from semiarid grasslands to extreme desert.

Pocket mice feed on a variety of seeds, green plant materials and some insects. Most actively store hoards of seeds in their burrows. Most species can survive for long periods without water, and some, at least, thrive in captivity for weeks at a time on a diet of dry seeds. They make up for a lack of water by reabsorbing water from their kidney wastes and produce water as part of their normal metabolism.

They also keep cool by regulating their body temperature by their behavior. They spend daylight hours and even hot, dry nights in underground burrows where the temperature is lower and the relative humidity is higher. Winter months are spent in hibernation.

Three major types of pocket mice can be recognized: kangaroo mice, spiny pocket mice and silky pocket mice.

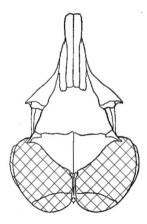

Top view of Skull of Kangaroo rat, showing extremely inflated auditory bullae (cross-hatched areas).

Kangaroo Mice

Only two kinds of this small, soft-haired mouse are known. They are restricted to desert habitats in Nevada and some adjacent parts of California and Utah.

The kangaroo mouse looks like a cross between a small kangaroo rat and a pocket mouse. The head is large and wide and the external cheek pouches are fur-lined. The ears are small. Unlike kangaroo rats, kangaroo mice have a relatively short tail, covered with short hairs and with no tuft at the tip. The base of the tail is small, the middle is enlarged, and the tip is pointed. The soles of the feet are densely haired and edged with stiff, projecting hairs.

Measurements of representative adults include: total length, 6.7 in. (170mm); tail, 3.5 in. (90mm); hind foot, 1 in. (25mm); ear, 0.4 in. (10 mm); and weight, 0.4 oz. (12g).

Kangaroo mice prefer areas with loose, drifting sand at elevations between 3,900 (1,200m) and 7,600 feet (2,340m) in northern and central Nevada, western Utah, and eastern California.

They hibernate from late October to late March. Their diet includes various seeds, insects, and green plants. Two litters of two to seven young, usually four, are born, one in the spring and one in the summer.

Kangaroo mice have not been reported as reservoirs of any human diseases.

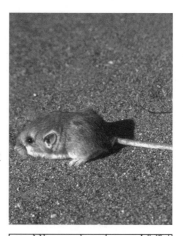

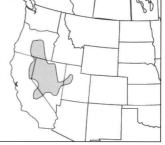

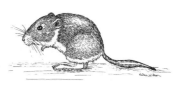

KANGAROO MICE,
Family Heteromyidae,
Subfamily Perognathinae,
genus *Microdipodops* (2 species)

Spiny Pocket Mice

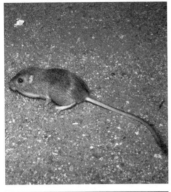

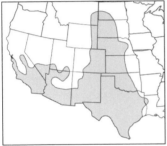

Spiny pocket mice are usually larger than their silky cousins. They are covered with a harsher fur that contains a number of obvious stiff hairs, some brownish, others whitish. The color of the back is darker, usually a grayish buff. The belly is whitish. The mouse's tail is longer than its head and body and has a weakly developed tuft of hairs at the tip. These mice have fur-lined cheek pouches.

Measurements of a typical adult include: total length, 8.2 in. (210mm); tail, 4.5 in. (115mm); hind foot, 1 in. (25mm); ear, 0.4 in. (10mm); and weight, 0.9 oz. (25g).

Spiny pocket mice occur in the grasslands and deserts of the western United States. They are active only at night from early spring to early fall and spend the cold months in hibernation. Their burrow is generally constructed under a bush or next to a rock. Their diet includes mostly seeds, but green vegetation and insects are also eaten.

Chagas' disease has been associated with spiny pocket mice.

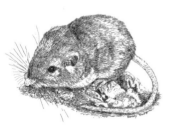

SPINY POCKET MICE,
Family Heteromyidae,
Subfamily Perognathinae,
genus *Chaetodipus* (9 species)

Silky Pocket Mice

Silky pocket mice are small, with a wide head, short neck, and tiny ears. They're covered with soft, light-colored fur, and have no stiff, spiny hairs. The tail is longer than the head and body and lacks a tuft of hair at the tip. The mouse has a well developed fur-lined cheek pouch on each side of the head.

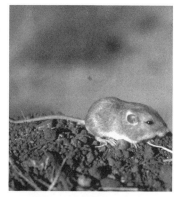

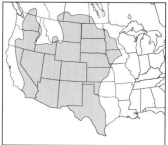

Measurements of a typical adult are: total length, 5.1 in. (130mm); tail, 2.1 in. (55mm); hind foot, 0.6 in. (18mm); ear, 0.2 in. (6mm); and weight, 0.3 oz. (8g).

Like their spiny relatives, silky pocket mice are common in sandy areas in desert grasslands, but they rarely occur in rocky deserts. They are active at night, from late spring to early fall, and spend the winter in hibernation. They feed mainly on the seeds of grasses and other small plants but also eat insects and some green plants, especially in the spring. They collect and transport seeds in their cheek pouches and store them in burrows.

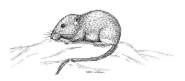

Silky pocket mice have not been associated with any of the diseases described in this book.

SILKY POCKET MICE,
Family Heteromyidae,
Subfamily Perognathinae,
genus *Perognathus* (9 species)

SUBFAMILY DIPODOMINAE — KANGAROO RATS

The second subfamily of desert rodents, the kangaroo rats, consists of only a single living genus. These rodents are highly modified for hopping. Their hind limbs and feet are much enlarged, the forelimbs are short, and the long tail has a large tuft of hair at the tip. The auditory bullae (see page 106) are extremely inflated, resulting in a large, wide head. Habitats range from grasslands to arid deserts.

Kangaroo Rats

Kangaroo rats have long, soft fur that is usually tan, buff, or cinnamon on the back. A white stripe runs across the thighs. The belly has long, soft, white hairs. The rat also has fur-lined external cheek pouches.

Measurements of a typical species include: total length, 9.8 in. (25 mm); tail, 5.9 in. (15 mm); hind foot, 1.5 in. (4 mm); ear, 0.5 in. (1 mm); and weight, 1.6 oz. (44g). Some larger species are almost twice this size.

Kangaroo rats live in a variety of habitats from grasslands to areas of soft, blowing sands. They are active at night, usually throughout the year. Their diet is mainly seeds. In times of surplus food, they collect seeds in their cheek pouches and store them in shallow holes in the ground or in their burrows. They also eat various insects and newly sprouted seeds.

Kangaroo rats have been found to serve as reservoirs in encephalitis, rabies and giardiasis.

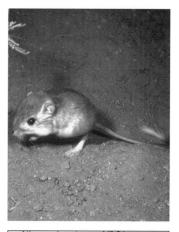

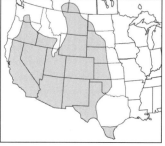

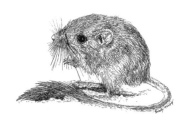

KANGAROO RATS,
Family Heteromyidae,
Subfamily Dipodominae,
genus *Dipodomys* (16 species)

Rats and Mice Family—
Muridae

The murids are, by far and away, the most abundant, widespread, and diversified rodent family. About 1,087 living species are recognized, grouped into 255 genera that are arranged in 17 subfamilies. This makes up about 65 percent of all living rodent species and about 26 percent of all living mammals. However, in the United States and Canada, the murid family is only slightly more diverse than the squirrel family.

Three Muridae subfamilies have representatives in this area: Sigmodontinae (New World rats and mice with 6 genera and 33 species here grouped in 6 major types), Arvicolinae (voles and lemmings with 5 genera and 16 species grouped in 2 major types), and Murinae (Old World rats and mice with 2 genera and 3 species grouped in 2 major types).

Subfamily Sigmodontinae
New World Rats and Mice

These rodents vary in size; length of the head and body can range from 50 to 360mm. This family includes the smallest living rodent, the pygmy mouse *(Baiomys)*. Among New World rats and mice, the tail may be either short or long, furred or naked. Most have a tail about the length of the head and body, with a slight tuft of hair at the tip. The limbs of these rodents also vary, ranging from short and stocky to long and slender.

These are the common rats and mice of much of North and South America. Most are herbivorous. Some specialize in feeding on grasses (graminivorous), others on seeds (granivorous), and still others feed on a wider variety of plant materials as well as various invertebrates. A few, such as the grasshopper mice *(Onychomys)*, feed almost entirely on insects. Habitats range from sea level to mountaintops, even within a single species (for example, one of the deer mice, *Peromyscus maniculatus,* shows this variation). Forests, grasslands and deserts are all inhabited by members of this family.

Rice Rat

About 55 species of rice rats are known. They range from the southeastern United States southward through Central America and most of South America. Only 2 species are known in the United States. They are slightly smaller than the Old World rats. Their tail is long and thinly haired.

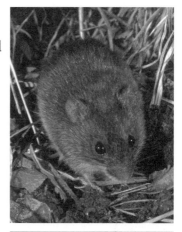

Measurements of a typical adult include: total length, 10 in. (25cn); tail, 5.5 in. (137mm); and weight, 2 oz. (57g).

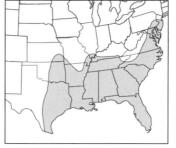

Rice rats live mainly in marshy areas where they can easily swim underwater. Food includes land and aquatic plants as well as fungi, insects and snails. Some are found in grassy areas away from water.

To date, no human diseases have been associated with rice rats in the United States.

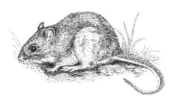

RICE RAT,
Family Muridae,
Subfamily Sigmodontinae,
genus *Oryzomys* (2 species)

Harvest Mice

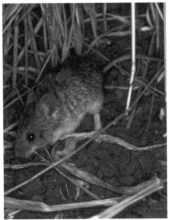

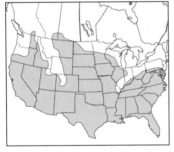

This small mouse has small ears, a long slender tail that is only sparsely haired, no external fur-lined cheek pouches, and a vertical groove on the front of each upper incisor. It is brownish above and white below. The sides have a line of buff-colored fur between the dorsal and ventral colors. Young are grey in color.

Measurements of a typical adult are: total length, 5.5 in. (140mm); tail, 2.6 in. (65mm); hind foot, 0.7 in. (17mm); ear, 0.5 in. (12mm); and weight, 0.5 oz. (12g).

Harvest mice prefer grassy areas, and are most numerous in grasslands and mountain meadows. They feed on seeds and plant growth. They are most active at night throughout the year. Their usual nest is made of grass at ground level or sometimes in a low bush.

Leptospirosis has been found in harvest mice.

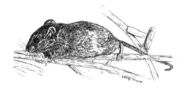

HARVEST MICE,
Family Muridae,
Subfamily Sigmodontinae,
genus *Reithrodontomys* (5 species)

Pygmy Mice

Smaller than a harvest mouse, this is the smallest known rodent now living. At first glance, it appears to be a young house mouse. However, the tail is shorter and hair-covered; the ears are small and rounded. The fur is dark gray, soft and shaggy. No groove is on the front surface of the upper incisors.

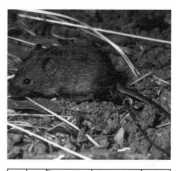

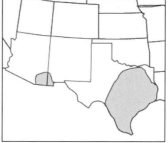

Measurements of a typical adult are: total length, 4.1 in. (105mm); tail, 1.8 in. (45mm); hind foot, 0.6 in. (14mm); ear, 0.4 in. (11mm); and weight, 0.4 oz. (10g).

In North America, pygmy mice are found in grasslands along the desert edge. They are active at night throughout the year, feeding mainly on grass shoots and some other green plant material.

Pygmy mice apparently don't serve as reservoirs of any human diseases in the United States.

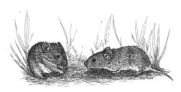

PYGMY MICE,
Family Muridae,
Subfamily Sigmodontinae,
Baiomys taylori,
Northern pygmy mouse

Deer Mice

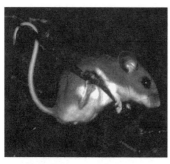

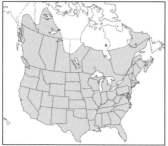

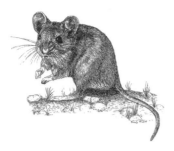

DEER MICE,
Family Muridae,
Subfamily Sigmodontinae,
genus *Peromyscus* (17 species)

Deer mice are similar to harvest mice in appearance, but are larger, especially in the length of the ears and the diameter of the tail. There is no groove on the front surface of the upper incisor. Colors vary from dark grayish to light buff-brown above, with white below. The tail is white with a narrow, distinct dark stripe on the dorsal surface. As with most members of this family, the young's first coat of fur is light gray.

Typical measurements for an adult are: total length, 7.1 in. (180mm); tail, 3.1 in. (80mm); hind foot, 0.9 in. (22mm); ear, 0.7 in. (17mm); and weight, 1 oz. (28g).

These mice are most commonly found in grasslands but also occur in small grassy areas surrounded by dense forests. Related species occur in almost all habitats in the United States, from sea level to mountaintops.

Deer mice are active at night throughout the year. They construct short underground burrows with nests of grasses or other soft material. Their diet includes insects and other arthropods but is mainly fungi, berries, fruits, small nuts, and seeds.

Deer mice have been found to serve as reservoirs for hanta virus pulmonary syndrome, Rocky Mountain spotted fever, leptospirosis, Lyme disease and plague.

Grasshopper Mice

These plump-bodied mice have short, thick tails and relatively short legs. The tail, less than half the length of the head and body, is constricted at the base. The back is generally pale cinnamon to light brown in color. The belly and feet are white.

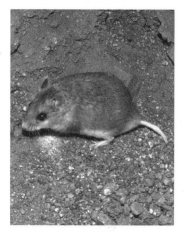

Measurements of a typical adult are: total length, 5.4 in. (138mm); tail, 1.6 in. (40mm); hind foot, 0.8 in. (20mm); ear, 0.7 in. (19mm); and weight, 1.2 oz. (35g).

Grasshopper mice live in grasslands where they are active at night throughout the year. They are more carnivorous than other small rodents. Their food consists mainly of invertebrates, especially grasshoppers—hence their common name. They hunt in small groups and have a high-pitched whistle that apparently helps keep the group together. Each group has a system of burrows, including a central nest burrow, which is closed during the day. They also build food-storage burrows to hold seeds for use when insects are not available, and a series of short escape burrows throughout the normal hunting territory.

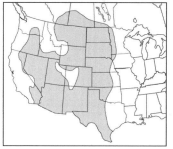

Grasshopper mice have not been implicated as reservoirs of any of the diseases in this area.

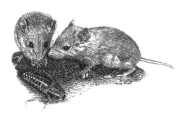

GRASSHOPPER MICE,
Family Muridae,
Subfamily Sigmodontinae,
genus *Onychomys* (2 species)

Cotton Rats

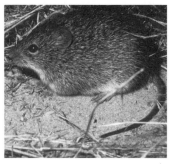

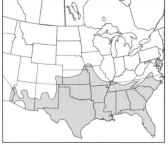

This small rat has coarsely grizzled, generally blackish or brownish fur with a mixture of buff or gray hairs. The sides and belly are lighter in color. The tail is shorter than the head and body.

Measurements of a typical adult are: total length, 9.8 in. (250mm); tail, 4.1 in. (105mm); hind foot, 1.3 in. (32mm); ear, 0.7 in. (17mm); and weight, 3.2 oz. (90g).

Cotton rats thrive in tall grasses and weed-grown fields. They are active throughout the year, often feeding during the day. They make runways along which they place small stacks of short grass stems. Food is mainly the stems and new growth of grasses and weeds.

Cotton rats serve as reservoirs of encephalitis, rabies, Rocky Mountain spotted fever, leptospirosis and Chagas' disease.

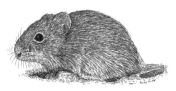

COTTON RATS,
Family Muridae,
Subfamily Sigmodontinae,
genus *Sigmodon* (4 species)

Wood Rats

Most wood rats have a thick, round, blunt-ended tail that is covered with short hairs and is shorter than the head and body. One species (the bushy-tailed wood rat) has a bushy squirrel-like tail. The ears are large and naked. The fur is soft, dense, and, on body and tail, and on both the body and tail is dark above and white below. Wood rats are also known as *pack rats;* they usually build a characteristic pile of sticks and other materials around nest sites. They are often found under a cactus or in a wood pile.

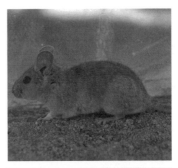

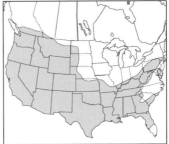

Measurements of a typical adult include: total length, 15.8 in. (400mm); tail, 5.1 in. (130mm); hind foot, 1.7 in. (52mm); ear, 1.4 in. (35mm); and weight, 10.6 oz. (300g).

Wood rats are found in a variety of habitats from sea level to high mountains. Some build their nests in crevices in rock ledges, or even in caves, mines, or abandoned buildings. They are active at night throughout the year. For food, they consume fungi and a wide variety of herbs, including stems and leaf shoots of trees, bushes, and cacti. Some insects are also eaten.

Wood rats have been found to serve as reservoirs for Lyme disease, plague and Chagas' disease.

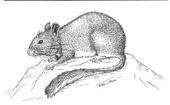

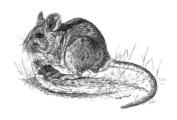

WOOD RATS,
Family Muridae,
Subfamily Sigmodontinae,
genus *Neotoma* (8 species)

Subfamily Arvicolinae — Lemmings and Voles

This subfamily of Muridae rats and mice includes about 87 living species (about 5 percent of all rodents), grouped into 18 genera. They are Holarctic in distribution, meaning they occur in northern regions of North America, Europe, and Asia, from sea level to high mountains. The lemmings are among the few terrestrial mammals that inhabit the extreme northern land masses. Two major types of this family can be recognized in this area: voles and muskrats.

Voles or Meadow Mice

These chunky-bodied, short-snouted mice have short ears; large, beadlike eyes; and long, loose, soft, grizzled fur. In most species, the fur on the back is dark in color but a few have a dorsal rusty or reddish stripe. The tail is usually short and sharply bicolored, dark above and white below. The limbs are short.

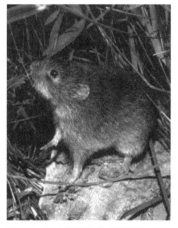

Most voles, also called *meadow mice,* live on the ground, mainly in grasses but some, like the *Phenacomys,* live mainly in trees. They are mostly active at night throughout the year. In areas with winter snow, they construct feeding tunnels under the snow.

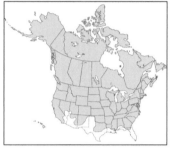

Measurements of a typical adult vole are: total length, 5.5 in. (140mm); tail, 1.4 in. (35mm); hind foot, 0.8 in. (18mm); ear, 0.6 in. (15mm); and weight, 1.3 oz. (37g).

Diseases that have been isolated from voles include Colorado tick fever, rabies, Rocky Mountain spotted fever, leptospirosis, murine typhus, plague, relapsing fever, tularemia and giardiasis.

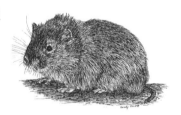

VOLES OR MEADOW MICE,
Family Muridae,
Subfamily Arvicolinae,
6 genera, 28 species

Muskrats

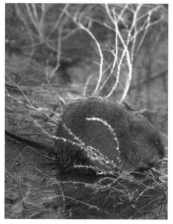

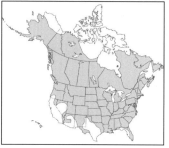

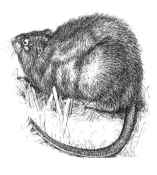

MUSKRATS,
Family Muridae,
Subfamily Arvicolinae,
Ondatra zibethicus, muskrat,
and *Neofiber alleni,*
round-tailed muskrat

Muskrats look like large meadow mice that are adapted for living in and near water. The typical muskrat has a scaly, flat, compressed tail that is about the same length as the head and body. The toes of the hind feet are fringed with stiff hairs that aid in swimming.

Round-tailed muskrats, slightly smaller than muskrats, live in Florida. Their tail is long, round, and fur-covered.

Measurements of a typical adult muskrat are: total length, 20 in. (500mm); tail, 10 in. (250mm); hind foot, 2.8 in. (72mm); ear, 0.8 in. (20mm); and weight, 4 pounds (1.8kg).

Muskrats live in and around permanent streams, lakes, and ponds in most of the United States, even up to elevations of 11,000 feet (3,354 m). They are active at night throughout the year, and eat any plant that grows in or near water. When available, muskrats eat crops such as corn. They create domed dens of vegetation and mud that rise above the water and have an entrance below water.

Diseases isolated from muskrats include rabies, intestinal bacteria, leptospirosis and tularemia.

Subfamily Murinae — Old World Rats and Mice

The many species of Old World rats and mice are widely distributed in the temperate and tropical parts of the Old World (mainly Europe and Asia). The 460 or so species, grouped in 117 genera, comprise about 30 percent of all rodents and about 12 percent of all mammals. Almost all these rodents are rat- or mouse-shaped, and they range in head and body length from 55 mm to over 400 mm. The tail is varied (short or long, furred or naked) but in most the tail is scantily haired and about the same length as the head and body.

Three species (house mouse, black rat, and Norway rat) have become commensals of man, meaning they eat food obtained from human activity. They've followed human migration from the Old World to the New World, including the American Southwest. These three species are the only members of the subfamily that occur in North America.

House Mice

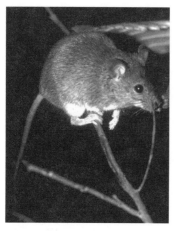

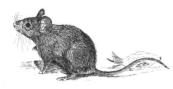

HOUSE MICE,
Family Muridae,
Subfamily Murinae,
species *Mus musculus,*
house mouse

House mice are well known to most people because they often live in human homes and other buildings. They're about the size and shape of harvest mice but their tails are long, scaly, hairless, and gray both above and below. The fur is usually grayish but sometime has a whitish or buff wash. The upper incisors are not grooved but have a distinctive notch in the grinding surface when viewed from the side.

Some varieties of house mice are used as pets and laboratory animals. Some of these are mutant house mice: albino (white), melanistic (black), and white with black "hoods."

Measurements of a typical adult include: total length, 6.7 in. (170mm); tail, 3.1 in. (80mm); hind foot, 0.7 in. (18mm); ear, 0.5 in. (12mm); and weight, 0.7 oz. (20g).

House mice rarely occur in undisturbed natural situations, but prefer to live in and around buildings and agricultural areas. They are adapted to living "with" human beings throughout most of the world, feeding on a varied diet, including crops, stored animal and human food, and insects. When food is available they can produce several (up to 14) litters of up to 16 young in a year. They make nests of soft material in hidden places: holes in the ground, in walls, under boards.

House mice have been associated with hanta virus pulmonary syndrome, leptospirosis, plague, intestinal bacteria and tularemia.

Old World Rats

These rats resemble the wood rat in general size but differ in having short ears and a sparsely haired, scaly tail that is slightly shorter than the head and body. The back, belly, and feet are grayish, with some brownish tones on the back. The white, black, and hooded rats found in pet stores and laboratories are often special varieties of these species.

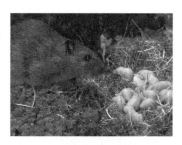

Measurements of a typical adult are: total length, 14.6 in. (370mm); tail, 6.7 in. (170mm); hind foot, 1.4 in. (35mm); ear, 0.9 in. (22mm); and weight, 10 oz. (280g).

These two rats are rarely found in undisturbed natural situations but they frequently occur in buildings, trash heaps, city dumps and other places that have been modified by humans. The Norway rat is widely distributed in both the U.S. and Canada. The black rat is generally found near coastlines, often in dock and pier areas. They now live with humans throughout most of the world, feeding on a wide variety of crops and stores of animal and human foods. Their reproductive rate is high: Adulthood is reached in 90 to 120 days. A litter contains from 2 to 20 young, and up to 9 litters are born in one year.

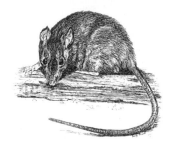

OLD WORLD RATS,
Family Muridae,
Subfamily Murinae,
Rattus norvegicus, Norway rat,
and *Rattus rattus,* black rat

These rats carry a series of human diseases, including Rocky Mountain spotted fever, leptospirosis, intestinal bacteria, plague, murine typhus and tularemia.

JUMPING MICE FAMILY AND RATS—DIPODIDAE

As currently understood, this family includes 37 species, grouped in 14 genera that are arranged in 6 subfamilies. Only one subfamily, Zapodinae, occurs in North America. It also includes a single genus and species known only in some isolated mountainous settings in China.

The family includes the jumping rats of the Old World deserts, the jerboas (27 species, arranged in 10 genera, 4 subfamilies), that are often extremely modified for jumping locomotion. Another subfamily, the birch mice, includes 5 species arranged in 3 genera. These mice have few modifications for jumping and occur only in birch forests of northern Eurasia.

Jumping Mice

These large mice have big hind feet, enlarged hind legs, and an elongated tail; all are adaptations for leaping. The upper incisors are grooved on the front surface. The back is dark, the sides yellowish or buff, the belly white. The ears are short and edged with light hairs. Unlike kangaroo rats and mice and pocket mice, jumping mice don't have externally opening fur-lined cheek pouches.

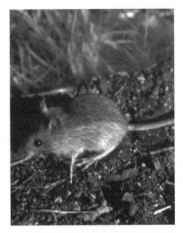

Measurements of a typical adult include: total length, 9.5 in. (240mm); tail, 5.7 in. (145mm); hind foot, 1.3 in. (32mm); ear, 0.6 in. (15mm); and weight, 0.8 oz. (23g).

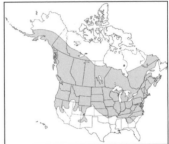

These animals become very fat in the fall, some gaining almost 25 percent of their body weight in the three weeks before entering hibernation.

In this area jumping mice are usually found in mountains in elevations from 4,000 to 11,000 feet (1,220-3,354m), especially under aspens and willows. They are active at night in the warmer parts of the year and hibernate during the cold months. Their nests are grass-lined structures in underground burrows.

Rocky Mountain spotted fever has been found in jumping mice.

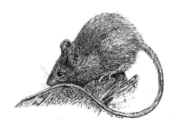

JUMPING MICE,
Family Dipodidae,
Subfamily Zapodinae,
2 genera, 4 species

PORCUPINE FAMILY — ERETHIZONTIDAE

Eight living species of porcupines, grouped in 3 genera, are known. They are natives of South America that invaded North America during the Pliocene epoch. The present distribution is not continuous, with one species occurring in the north-temperate areas of North America and the others restricted to tropical and subtropical regions of Central and South America.

Porcupines

This arboreal rodent is one of the largest known, larger than a small dog. It's well known for the spines (quills) found on its back, sides and tail. It is chunky-bodied with short legs. The claws (four on each front foot, five on the rear ones) are long and curved. The quills serve as protection from carnivores (bob cats, mountain lions, wolves) for these large, slow-moving rodents.

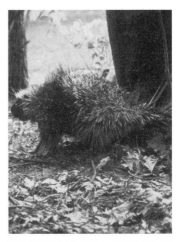

Measurements of a typical adult include: total length, 35 in. (890mm); tail, 8.3 in. (210mm); hind foot, 4.3 in. (110m); ear, 1.2 in. (30mm); and weight, 18 pounds (8.2kg).

Porcupines are most common in evergreen forests but in North America they're found almost anywhere there are trees, from sea level to above the timberline. They are generally active at night throughout the year, feeding on a variety of plants. Trees and bushes with the bark stripped from the trunks and branches are noticeable signs that porcupines are present, especially in the winter. They also eat twigs, leaves, stems of various trees, and herbs.

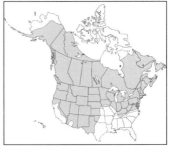

Porcupines are usually solitary and have a den in a cave, crevice or hollow tree. After a gestation period of about 120 days a single young (sometimes twins) is born, usually in late spring.

Diseases that have been isolated from porcupines include Colorado tick fever and tularemia.

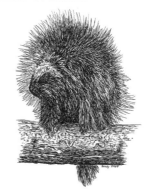

PORCUPINES,
Family Erethizontidae,
species *erethizon dorsatum,*
porcupine

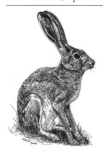

RABBITS AND PIKAS
(Order Lagomorpha)

Rabbits are native to all of the continents except Antarctica and Australia. The European rabbit was introduced into Australia and, once established, became a major pest. The order includes about 80 living species that are arranged in 13 genera in 2 families—the pikas, and the hares and rabbits.

All rabbits have four upper incisors; two of them are small "pegs" hidden behind the two large ones. Both the two large upper incisors and the two lower incisors are ever-growing. The diet of rabbits includes a number of different plants.

Pika Family (Ochotonidae)

These are small animals, about the size of a guinea pig. They have short ears, short legs, and a short tail hidden by fur. They include about 26 living species arranged in 2 genera, and occur in western North America and northeastern Asia. Pikas are generally restricted to rocky areas and, especially in the southern part of their range, to high mountains. Two species occur in the United States and Canada.

Pikas

Pikas have the general appearance of small cottontail rabbits but with short ears and no tail. The upper parts are grayish to buff in color. The underparts are lighter and are washed with buff.

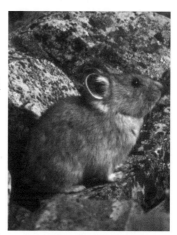

Average adult measurements are: total length, 8 in. (200mm); tail, 0.6 in. (16mm); hind foot, 1.2 in. (30mm); ear, 1 in. (25mm); and weight, 4.4 oz. (125g).

Rock exposure areas and slopes appear to be favorite habitats. Pikas are most active in early mornings and late afternoons throughout the year. They often sun on a rock, even at temperatures below freezing.

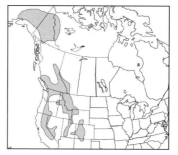

Food includes a variety of green vegetation. During the summer they harvest selected plants and spread them on rocks in the sunlight to cure as hay. In threatening weather the pikas move the drying hay under rocks, out of the rain. Once cured, the hay is stored under rocks and provides food for the winter season. They breed during the summer, and after a gestation period of 30 days a litter of two to five young is born. Two litters each summer are common.

Because the pikas live at high altitudes, there is little interaction with humans. Therefore, little testing has been done for diseases. No diseases are known to be transmitted by pikas.

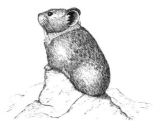

PIKAS,
Order Lagomorpha,
Family Ochotonidae

Hare and Rabbit Family (Leporidae)

This family includes about 54 species grouped into 11 genera. All rabbits and hares have hind limbs that are much longer than the forelimbs. Their ears are usually very long, always longer than wide. The tail is short but well-haired and quite evident. The females are larger than the males.

One of the smallest is the pygmy rabbit of the northwestern United States, which weighs only 0.55 lb. (250g). One of the largest, the antelope jackrabbit of the Southwest, can weigh up to 9 lb. (4.08kg).

Cottontails

Eight different species of cottontails occur in the United States and Canada. They are medium-sized and have relatively short ears, the inner surfaces of which are densely haired.

Measurements of a typical adult are: total length, 15.6 in. (400mm); tail, 1.3 in. (34mm); hind foot, 4 in. (100mm); ear, 2.4 in. (62mm); and weight, 2.5 pounds (1.1kg).

Although most cottontails live in brush, they also occur in a variety of habitats ranging from swamps and marshes to open grasslands. They feed on various grasses, herbs and other green vegetation. They're most active in the early morning and late evening, and at night during the summer.

After a gestation of about four weeks, the young are born in the warmer months. Three or four litters, each consisting of four to seven young, are born in an underground fur-lined nest. At birth the young are hairless, blind, and helpless. Maturity is reached nine to ten months after birth.

Diseases include rabies and, especially, tularemia and Rocky Mountain spotted fever.

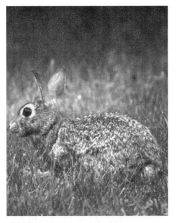

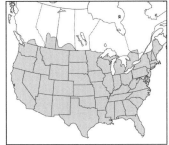

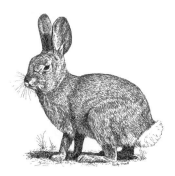

COTTONTAILS,
Order Lagomorpha,
Family Leporidae,
genus *Sylvilagus* (8 species)

Hares and Jackrabbits

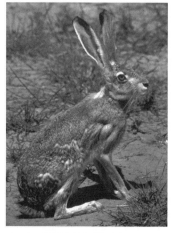

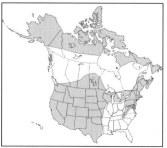

Six different members of this genus occur in the United States and Canada. Snowshoe hares are usually found in northern areas or in higher mountains of the West. Some populations become white in the winter. Jackrabbits are residents of the plains, grasslands, and deserts of the West.

Hares and jackrabbits usually have large hind legs and big ears. The upper parts of the body are grayish, the belly and tail white.

Measurements of a typical adult include: total length, 22.6 in. (575mm); tail, 3.2 in. (80mm); hind foot, 5.7 in. (145mm); ear, 4.3 in. (110mm); and weight, 5.7 pounds (2.5kg).

The young are precocial (born fully haired and with open eyes), and are able to follow their mother within a few minutes after birth.

Diseases include tularemia and Rocky Mountain spotted fever.

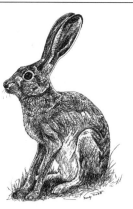

JACKRABBITS,
Order Lagomorpha,
Family Leporidae,
genus *Lepus* (6 species)

Some Useful References

The following references may be interesting to those who wish to learn more about bats, rodents, rabbits, and animal-borne diseases.

As already indicated, novices should seek professional advice from medical doctors concerning diseases. For general information concerning the identification and control of animals, consult state, provincial or federal wildlife biologists or agricultural extension agents. You can find phone numbers for these officials in the government offices section of the telephone directory. Professional pest-control technicians are the best sources for information about traps, poisons, and other control techniques.

Some references listed here are probably available at your nearest bookstore. Others are available in public libraries. Some of the more technical and out-of-print references may be found in major university libraries.

References About Diseases

References marked with an asterisk (*) are fairly elementary while those marked with two asterisks (**) are quite technical.

A number of excellent references exist about the various animal-borne diseases covered in this book. One of the most useful is the American Medical Association Encyclopedia of Medicine. Most standard encyclopedias have useful information listed under the name of the disease.

*Clayman, C.B., editor. 1989. *The American Medical Association Encyclopedia of Medicine.* Random House.

Some technical references about bat rabies are:

**Brass, D.A. 1994. *Rabies in Bats. Natural History and Public Health Implications.* Ridgefield, Conn.: Livia Press.

**Burnett, C.D. 1989. Bat rabies in Illinois, United States of America. *Journal of Wildlife Disease* 25(1):10-19.

**Childs, J.E., C.V. Trimorebi, and J.W. Krebs. 1994. The Epidemiology of Bat Rabies in New York State, 1988-1992. *Epidemiology and Infection,* 113 (3): 501-511.

**Krebs, John W., Tara W. Strine, Jean S. Smith, Charles E.Rupprecht, and James E. Childs. 1995. Rabies surveillance in the United States during 1994. *Journal of American Veterinary Medical Association* 207(12):1562-75.

**Warrell, Mary J. Human deaths from cryptic bat rabies in the United States of America. *Lancet* 346(8967):65. This is a brief summary of recent technical studies and reports concerning bat rabies.

References About Mammals

*Burt, William H., and R.P. Grossenheider. 1976, third edition. *A Field Guide to the Mammals.* New York: Houghton Mifflin.

*Cockrum, E. Lendell. 1982. *Mammals of the Southwest.* Tucson, Arizona: University of Arizona Press.

*Cockrum, E. Lendell, and Yar Petryszyn. 1993. *Mammals of the Southwestern United States and Northwestern Mexico.* Tucson, Ariz.: Treasure Chest Publications.

*Cockrum, E. Lendell, and Yar Petryszyn. 1994. *Mammals of California and Nevada.* Tucson, Ariz.: Treasure Chest Publications.

**Hall, E. Raymond. 1981, second edition, 2 vols. *The Mammals of North America.* New York: John Wiley & Sons.

**Jones, J. Knox Jr., Robert S. Hoffman, Dale W. Rice, Clyde Jones, Robert J. Baker, and Mark D. Engstrom. 1992. *Revised Checklist of North American Mammals North of Mexico, 1991.* Occasional Papers, The Museum, Texas Tech University, No. 146:1-23.

*Tuttle, Merlin D. 1988. *America's Neighborhood Bats.* Austin: University of Texas Press.

*Whitaker, John O. Jr. 1980. *The Audubon Society Field Guide to North American Mammals.* New York: Alfred A. Knopf.

**Wilson, Don E., and DeeAnn M. Reeder, editors. 1993, second edition. *Mammal Species of the World, A Taxonomic and Geographic Reference.* Washington: Smithsonian Institution.

Acknowledgments

First and foremost, I wish to thank my wife, Irma, for her continued tolerance of my wandering trips to libraries and for the asocial hours I spent at my word processor. Irma accompanied me as I visited many of the central and southeastern states that were not already known to me.

Special acknowledgments and thanks are due to those who contributed to the illustrations.

Most of the line drawings of mammals were made by Sandy Truett before her budding career as a wildlife artist was tragically ended in an automobile accident. I used these earlier in three handbooks (published by the University of Arizona Press or Treasure Chest Publications, Tucson, Arizona) listed in the references. Helen A. Wilson and Dr. Yar Petryszyn prepared others.

All of the bat photographs are the work of a former student of mine, Dr. Bruce Hayward, now retired from Western New Mexico State University. Those illustrated here are listed by common and scientific names: ghost-faced bat *(Mormoops megalophylla)*; short-eared, nectar-feeding, leaf-nosed bat *(Choeronycteris mexicana)*; big-eared, insect-feeding, leaf-nosed bat *(Macrotus californicus)*; mouse-eared bat *(Myotis thysanoides)*; pipistrelle *(Pipistrellus hesperus)*; silver-haired bat *(Lasionycteris noctivigans)*; hoary bat *(Lasiurus cinereus)*; red bat *(Lasiurus borealis)*; big-eared bat *(Plecotus townsendii)*; spotted bat *(Euderma maniculatum)*; Allen's big-eared bat *(Idionycteris phyllotis)*; pallid bat *(Antrozous pallidus)*; Brazilian free-tailed *(guano)* bat *(Tadarida brasiliensis)*; large free-tailed bat *(Nyctinomops femorosaccus)*; mastiff bat *(Eumops underwoodi)*.

Most of the photographs of rodents and all those of hares and rabbits were provided by the Mammal Slide Library of the American Society of Mammalogists. Dr. Elmer J. Finck,

Division of Biological Sciences, Emporia State University, Emporia, Kansas, is currently in charge of this library. The photographers and their photographs are: T.L. Best: antelope ground squirrel *(Ammospermophilus harrisii)*; silky pocket mouse *(Perognathus flavus)*; hares and jackrabbits *(Lepus californicus)*. L. Elliot: chipmunks *(Tamias striatus)*. R.B. Forbes: grasshopper mouse *(Onychomys leucogaster)*; vole and meadow mouse *(Microtus ochrogaster)*; muskrat *(Ondatra zibethicus)*. D.C. Huckaby: kangaroo mouse *(Microdipodops megacephalus)*; beaver *(Castor canadensis)*; wood rat *(Neotoma lepida)*; jumping mouse *(Zapus princeps)*. J. des Lauriers: pika *(Ochotona princeps)*. R.K. LaVal: rice rat *(Oryzomys palustris)*. L.L. Master: red squirrel *(Tamiasciurus hudsonicus)*; deer mouse *(Peromyscus leucopus)*; house mouse *(Mus musculus)*. G.C. Rinker: harvest mouse *(Reithrodontomys megalotis)*. V.C. Scheffer: mountain beaver *(Aplodontia rufa)*. E.J. Taylor: Old World rat *(Rattus norvegicus)*. G.L. Twiest: marmot *(Marmota monax)*; tree squirrel *(Sciurus niger)*; porcupine *(Erethizon dorsatum)*; cottontail *(Sylvilagus floridanus)*. N.M. Wells: flying squirrel *(Glaucomys volans)*.

Two associates of mine at the University of Arizona provided the following photographs: Dr. Yar Petryszyn of the Department of Ecology and Evolutionary Biology: spiny pocket mouse *(Chaetodipus penicillatus)*; pocket gopher *(Thomomys bottae)*; ground squirrel *(Spermophilus tereticaudus)*. Dr. Cecil Schwabe of the Department of Renewable Natural Resources: prairie dog *(Cynomys ludovicianus)*; kangaroo rat *(Dipodomys spectabilis)*; pygmy mouse *(Baiomys taylori)*; cotton rat *(Sigmodon ochrognathus)*.

Anita Alsup-Page and Rachel Carmichael converted my sketches of distribution into publishable maps.

Personnel at Fisher Books converted some data into graphs and prepared the final distribution maps which were then converted into computer artwork by Miriam Fisher. Bill Fisher, especially, should be acknowledged for his extensive editorial efforts.

My great thanks to all.

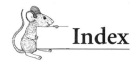

Index